HEALTH CARE IN TRANSITION

DEFENSE HEALTH CARE

TREATMENT, PERFORMANCE AND TRICARE

HEALTH CARE IN TRANSITION

Additional books and e-books in this series can be found on Nova's website under the Series tab.

HEALTH CARE IN TRANSITION

DEFENSE HEALTH CARE

TREATMENT, PERFORMANCE AND TRICARE

FREDERICK DUNCAN
EDITOR

snova
New York

Library of Congress Cataloging-in-Publication Data

ISBN: 978-1-53615-175-6

Published by Nova Science Publishers, Inc. † New York

CONTENTS

Preface		**vii**
Chapter 1	Defense Health Care: Expanded Use of Quality Measures Could Enhance Oversight of Provider Performance *United States Government Accountability Office*	**1**
Chapter 2	Defense Health Care: DOD Should Demonstrate How Its Plan to Transfer the Administration of Military Treatment Facilities Will Improve Efficiency *United States Government Accountability Office*	**43**
Chapter 3	Defense Health Care: Additional Assessments Needed to Better Ensure an Efficient Total Workforce *United States Government Accountability Office*	**83**
Chapter 4	Defense Health Care: TRICARE Surveys Indicate Nonenrolled Beneficiaries' Access to Care Has Generally Improved *United States Government Accountability Office*	**145**

Chapter 5 Defense Health Care:
Tricare Select Implementation Plan Included Mandated Elements, But Access Standards Should Be Clarified **181**
United States Government Accountability Office

Index **201**

PREFACE

For over a decade, Congress and DOD have led a series of efforts to address the governance structure of the Military Health System. In chapter1, GAO examines (1) measures DOD uses to assess the quality of direct and purchased care, and (2) the extent to which DOD has established performance standards related to the measures and corrective action requirements for providers who do not meet those standards. As reported in chapter 2, or more than a decade, partially in response to congressional mandates, DOD has worked to address inefficiencies in the Military Health System to control costs. Chapter 3 examines the military departments' planning processes for determining (1) operational medical personnel requirements, including an assessment of the mix of federal civilian, contractor, and active and reserve medical personnel; and (2) the most appropriate workforce mix at MTFs and any challenges in executing their desired workforce mix. The National Defense Authorization Act (NDAA) for Fiscal Year 2008 directed DOD to conduct surveys of nonenrolled beneficiaries and civilian providers about access to care under the TRICARE Standard and Extra options. It also directed GAO to review the surveys' results. Additionally, the NDAA for Fiscal Year 2017 included a provision for GAO to review access to care under TRICARE Extra. Chapter 4 addresses both provisions. The NDAA 2017 made several changes to the TRICARE program, including the establishment of a new preferred provider network health plan option called TRICARE Select. The NDAA 2017 made several changes to the TRICARE program, including the establishment of a new preferred provider network health plan option called TRICARE Select. GAO examined program policies, procedures, and contracts and interviewed DOD officials and TRICARE regional contractors as reported in chapter 5.

Chapter 1 - The National Defense Authorization Act for fiscal year 2016 contains provisions for GAO to review DOD's plans to (1) improve the experience of beneficiaries who receive care through military hospitals and clinics or from civilian providers and (2) reduce variation in the quality of care. In this chapter, GAO examines (1) measures DOD uses to assess the quality of direct and purchased care, and (2) the extent to which DOD has established performance standards related to the measures and corrective action requirements for providers who do not meet those standards. GAO reviewed the measures in DOD's Core Dashboard for direct care and Purchased Care Dashboard for purchased care. It also reviewed DOD documents and reports to Congress, and interviewed MHS officials, including officials from the Army, Navy, and Air Force. GAO also compared the quality measures DOD uses to those used in Medicare and by private insurers, which have been vetted by multiple stakeholders. GAO assessed DOD's use of performance standards and corrective action requirements in the context of federal internal control standards.

Chapter 2 - In fiscal year 2017, DOD provided health care to 9.4 million beneficiaries, including service members, retirees, and their families at a cost of $43 billion. For more than a decade, partially in response to congressional mandates, DOD has worked to address inefficiencies in the Military Health System to control costs. To further achieve efficiencies, the NDAA for Fiscal Year 2017 required DOD to develop an implementation plan that addressed four elements related to transferring the administration of the MTFs to the DHA. DOD issued the plan in June 2018. The NDAA also included a provision for GAO to review the plan. GAO determined whether (1) DOD's plan included the statutory elements related to the transfer of administration of the MTFs to the DHA and (2) additional information would be useful to demonstrate that the plan will reduce or better manage duplication and improve efficiencies. GAO assessed DOD's plan against the required elements and, where appropriate, considered the extent to which the plan provided detailed information related to key change management practices identified in past GAO work.

Chapter 3 - The MHS includes more than 241,000 active duty, reserve, federal civilian, and contractor personnel who provide (1) operational medical care in support of war and other contingencies and (2) beneficiary medical care within DOD's hospitals and clinics. The Senate Report 115-125 accompanying a bill for the National Defense Authorization Act for Fiscal Year 2018 contained a provision for GAO to review how DOD determines its mix of military, federal civilian, and contractor personnel. This chapter examines the military departments' planning processes for determining (1) operational medical personnel requirements, including an assessment of the mix of federal civilian, contractor, and active and reserve medical personnel; and (2) the most appropriate workforce mix at MTFs and any challenges in executing their desired workforce mix. GAO compared MHS staffing practices with DOD policy, and analyzed fiscal year 2017 budgetary data to determine the proportion of military, federal civilian, and contractor personnel. GAO also interviewed senior leaders at six MTFs.

Chapter 4 - DOD provides health care, including mental health care, to eligible beneficiaries through TRICARE. Beneficiaries who use TRICARE Prime, a managed care option, must enroll to receive care. Prior to Jan. 1, 2018, beneficiaries did not need to enroll for TRICARE Standard, a fee- for-service option, or TRICARE Extra, a preferred provider organization option (referred to as nonenrolled beneficiaries). Although the TRICARE Standard and Extra options were terminated effective Jan. 1, 2018, the new TRICARE Select option has similar benefits for obtaining care from network and non-network providers. The National Defense Authorization Act (NDAA) for Fiscal Year 2008 directed DOD to conduct surveys of nonenrolled beneficiaries and civilian providers about access to care under the TRICARE Standard and Extra options. It also directed GAO to review the surveys' results. Additionally, the NDAA for Fiscal Year 2017 included a provision for GAO to review access to care under TRICARE Extra. This chapter addresses both provisions. GAO analyzed DOD's surveys to determine (1) nonenrolled beneficiaries' access to care, (2) nonenrolled beneficiaries' ratings of TRICARE, (3) civilian providers' awareness and acceptance of TRICARE, and (4) nonenrolled beneficiaries' access by individual geographic area. GAO interviewed agency officials, analyzed the 2012-2015 surveys, and compared them to DOD's 2008-2011 surveys and to surveys of Medicare and Medicaid beneficiaries. In commenting on a draft of this chapter, DOD concurred with GAO's findings.

Chapter 5 - DOD offers health care services to approximately 9.4 million eligible beneficiaries through TRICARE, DOD's regionally structured health care program. In each of its regions, DOD uses contractors to manage health care delivery through civilian provider networks, among other tasks. The NDAA 2017 made several changes to the TRICARE program, including the establishment of a new preferred provider network health plan option called TRICARE Select. The NDAA 2017 also required DOD to develop an implementation plan for TRICARE Select that addresses seven specific mandated elements on access to care, beneficiary complaints, and quality metrics for network providers. The NDAA 2017 included a provision for GAO to review the implementation plan. This chapter examines the extent to which DOD's implementation plan addressed the mandated elements. GAO evaluated DOD's implementation plan using leading planning practices identified in GAO's prior work and standards for internal control. GAO examined program policies, procedures, and contracts and interviewed DOD officials and TRICARE regional contractors.

In: Defense Health Care
Editor: Frederick Duncan

ISBN: 978-1-53615-175-6

Chapter 1

DEFENSE HEALTH CARE: EXPANDED USE OF QUALITY MEASURES COULD ENHANCE OVERSIGHT OF PROVIDER PERFORMANCE*

United States Government Accountability Office

ABBREVIATIONS

CLABSI	central line-associated bloodstream infection
CMS	Centers for Medicare & Medicaid Services
CQMC	Core Quality Measures Collaborative
DHA	Defense Health Agency
DOD	Department of Defense
HEDIS	Healthcare Effectiveness Data and Information Set
MHS	Military Health System

* This is an edited, reformatted and augmented version of United States Government Accountability Office; Report to Congressional Committees; Accessible Version, Publication No. GAO-18-574, dated September 2018.

MTF	military treatment facility
NDAA	National Defense Authorization Act
P4I	Partnership for Improvement

WHY GAO DID THIS STUDY

The National Defense Authorization Act for fiscal year 2016 contains provisions for GAO to review DOD's plans to (1) improve the experience of beneficiaries who receive care through military hospitals and clinics or from civilian providers and (2) reduce variation in the quality of care.

In this chapter, GAO examines (1) measures DOD uses to assess the quality of direct and purchased care, and (2) the extent to which DOD has established performance standards related to the measures and corrective action requirements for providers who do not meet those standards.

GAO reviewed the measures in DOD's Core Dashboard for direct care and Purchased Care Dashboard for purchased care. It also reviewed DOD documents and reports to Congress, and interviewed MHS officials, including officials from the Army, Navy, and Air Force. GAO also compared the quality measures DOD uses to those used in Medicare and by private insurers, which have been vetted by multiple stakeholders. GAO assessed DOD's use of performance standards and corrective action requirements in the context of federal internal control standards.

WHAT GAO RECOMMENDS

The MHS should (1) prioritize, as appropriate, selecting quality measures common for both direct and purchased care that expand the range of quality areas covered by the measures and (2) establish consistent performance standards and corrective action requirements for direct and purchased care providers. DOD concurred with both recommendations.

WHAT GAO FOUND

The National Defense Authorization Act for fiscal year 2016 (NDAA 2016) directed the Department of Defense (DOD) to align its measures of health care quality used in the Military Health System (MHS) to improve beneficiary experience and reduce variation in the quality of care. GAO reviewed the quality measures DOD identified in March 2017 in response to the NDAA 2016; DOD senior leadership tracks these measures on dashboards to gauge progress on MHS strategic goals. GAO found that DOD does not use a common set of measures on its dashboards to assess the quality of care provided by either military hospitals and clinics—known as direct care—or networks of civilian hospitals and other providers, known as purchased care (See Figure 2, p21). As a result, DOD's senior leadership has limited information on the extent to which MHS beneficiaries receive consistently high quality care across the MHS.

Furthermore, for both direct and purchased care, DOD uses measures on its dashboards that track a limited range of quality care areas and medical conditions compared to the measures adopted by Medicare and by private health insurers. For example, whereas civilian hospitals report to Medicare information on 11 measures of patients' self-reported experience in hospitals, Military hospitals report only 1 such measure. By using a limited range of quality measures, DOD may not detect key quality issues. Further, when selecting quality measures, the MHS does not prioritize using common measures across direct and purchased care or expanding the range of measures it uses.

GAO also found that for direct care DOD has established performance standards and corrective action requirements for military hospitals or clinics that do not meet those standards in direct care. The performance standards indicate the level of performance providers should meet on the various quality measures DOD tracks on its dashboards, and the corrective action requirements instruct providers to take steps to improve care. However, for purchased care, DOD has not established similar performance standards for individual providers. Without consistent performance standards and corrective action requirements, DOD is limited in its ability to address variation in the quality of care delivered and help ensure that its beneficiaries receive consistent high quality care across the MHS.

September 17, 2018

The Honorable Jim Inhofe
Chairman

The Honorable Jack Reed
Ranking Member
Committee on Armed Services
United States Senate

The Honorable Mac Thornberry
Chairman

The Honorable Adam Smith
Ranking Member
Committee on Armed Services
House of Representatives

The Department of Defense's (DOD) Military Health System (MHS) offers a full range of health care services to over 9 million eligible beneficiaries, including active duty servicemembers and their dependents, medically-eligible National Guard and Reserve members and their dependents, and retirees and their dependents and survivors, among others. These beneficiaries may receive care from military treatment facilities (MTFs)— known as direct care—or from civilian hospitals, physicians, and other clinicians participating in DOD-sponsored health plans that are administered by contractors—known as purchased care.[1] While MTFs take

[1] The program through which the MHS administers these health care services using direct and purchased care providers is called TRICARE. DOD reported that for fiscal year 2018, the direct care providers included 51 inpatient hospitals and medical centers located at military installations distributed across the U.S. and abroad, plus another 381 ambulatory care clinics

the lead in delivering health care to active duty servicemembers, eligible beneficiaries can receive a wide array of primary and specialty care from the MTFs, purchased care providers, or both. Overall, about 60 percent of all the health care services that beneficiaries received in 2017 were delivered through purchased care.

In 2014, the Secretary of Defense ordered a comprehensive review of the MHS that found considerable variation in the quality of care delivered. For example, the review found that 8 of 17 MTFs with high volume surgery programs had higher than expected rates of surgical complications. Furthermore, in the case of purchased care, the review found that DOD had limited information on the quality of care delivered by those civilian providers.[2]

The information DOD has on the quality of care in the MHS comes from what it collects on various quality measures. In general, health care quality measures are standard, evidence based metrics—such as the percentage of patients receiving a screening or the rate of hospital readmissions or surgical complications—that health care systems such as the MHS use to quantify health care processes, outcomes, and other aspects of care. Health care quality measures can be linked to performance standards established for providers. For example, a quality measure may indicate the percentage of patients who receive a diabetes screening, while a related performance standard may be that providers are expected to ensure that at least a certain percentage of applicable patients receive the screening each year.

Section 730 of the National Defense Authorization Act for Fiscal Year 2016 (NDAA 2016) directed DOD to develop plans to enhance the experience of beneficiaries receiving care under the MHS and eliminate variation in the quality of care that beneficiaries receive across direct and purchased care. The Act stipulated that DOD align the measures used to assess the quality of direct and purchased care to improve care across the MHS as a whole.[3] In March 2017, DOD issued its response to section 730,

---

and 247 dental clinics. There are 3,664 civilian hospitals, over 600,000 civilian clinicians, and over 76,000 dentists participating in the MHS's purchased care networks.

[2] Department of Defense, *Final Report to the Secretary of Defense, Military Health System Review* (August 2014).

[3] Pub. L. No. 114-92, § 730(a), 129 Stat. 726, 874 (2015).

reporting that it had established two sets of quality measures— a set of measures for direct care described as "core measures" and another set of measures for purchased care. The MHS reported to Congress that the core direct care measures and purchased care measures are the key quality measures DOD's senior health care leadership use to track DOD's progress towards achieving the department's overall strategic goals of providing high quality care across the MHS as a whole.[4] DOD reported that it aligned these quality measures across direct and purchased care where possible.[5]

Section 730 of the NDAA 2016 also includes a provision for us to assess the strengths and limitations of DOD's plans for achieving the Act's objectives.[6] In this chapter, we examine

1) the core direct care measures and purchased care measures DOD uses to assess the quality of care in the MHS; and
2) the extent to which DOD has established performance standards related to its core direct care measures and purchased care measures and corrective action requirements for providers that do not meet these performance standards.

To examine the core direct care measures and purchased care measures DOD uses to assess the quality of care in the MHS, we focused our review on the measures listed on the Core Dashboard and Purchased Care Dashboard, which are used in direct care and purchased care, respectively.[7] We focused on the dashboard measures because the MHS reported to Congress that these are the measures that DOD health care leaders rely on

---

[4] DOD describes these overall strategic goals for the MHS as its "Quadruple Aim": improved readiness, better health, better care, and lower cost. This builds on the "Triple Aim" widely adopted by civilian health care providers, with the addition of readiness.

[5] U.S. Department on Defense, *Response to Section 730 of the National Defense Authorization Act for Fiscal Year 2016 (Public Law 114-92): Report on Plans to Improve Experience with and Eliminate Performance Variability of Health Care Provided by the Department of Defense*, Mar. 13, 2017.

[6] Pub. L. No. 114-92, § 730(b), 129 Stat. 726, 874 (2015).

[7] Officials told us and our review of MHS documents confirmed that the MHS tracks other quality measures not on the dashboards as part of various initiatives for direct care, and the MHS's purchased care contractors monitor quality measures as part of their quality improvement activities. These measures were outside the scope of our review.

to establish accountability throughout the MHS and identify areas where quality improvement is needed. The measures on the dashboards are periodically updated, and we examined the measures included on the dashboards as of March 31, 2018 and the extent to which the measures on one dashboard aligned with those on the other. We also examined the range of quality care areas and medical conditions assessed by the dashboard measures and compared these to the range of quality care areas and medical conditions assessed by the measures included in the Hospital Compare measure set for inpatient care and the Core Quality Measure Collaborative (CQMC) measure sets for outpatient care.[8] Because the Hospital Compare and CQMC measures for inpatient and outpatient care have been vetted and reviewed by multiple health care stakeholders and widely adopted, we determined that they represented appropriate benchmarks for assessing the scope of the MHS's quality assessment.[9] We also reviewed DOD documents to understand DOD senior health leadership's decisions to select and track the measures on the Core and Purchased Care Dashboards and not others. Specifically, we systematically reviewed minutes from 335 meetings of the MHS governance bodies—which represent the three military services that provide health care services under the MHS (Army, Navy, and Air Force) and other components of the MHS—that make final decisions on the measures to be included on the Core and Purchased Care Dashboards.[10] We

---

[8] The Hospital Compare website provides publicly available information on the quality of care at hospitals and is maintained by the Centers for Medicare & Medicaid Services (CMS). The website can be found at https://www.medicare.gov/hospitalcompare/search.html, accessed on May 1, 2018. The CQMC is a multi-stakeholder voluntary effort on quality measure alignment that includes representatives from CMS, major private health insurers, and medical specialty societies. The CQMC has developed multiple measure sets for outpatient care—the CQMC measure sets—which are available at https://www.cms.gov/Medicare/Quality-InitiativesPatient-Assessment-Instruments/QualityMeasures/Core-Measures.html, accessed on May 1, 2018.

[9] Hospital Compare, and to a lesser extent, the CQMC measure sets, have been widely adopted by 4,000 Medicare hospitals and by major private insurers to assess the quality of inpatient and outpatient care.

[10] These governance bodies are the Senior Military Medical Action Council, the Medical Deputies Action Group, and the Medical Operations Group, which each include representatives from the Army, Navy, and Air Force. The Navy also provides health care services for the Marine Corps. We reviewed the minutes of these governance bodies for the period starting January 1, 2015, which coincided with the initiation of the MHS's Partnership for Improvement performance management system following the release of the MHS's 2014 comprehensive review. We completed our review on March 31, 2018.

supplemented this document review with interviews of the MHS officials responsible for managing direct care as well as those responsible for overseeing the MHS's contracting of purchased care. We also interviewed representatives of the medical commands for each of the three military services to obtain their perspectives on the measures that the MHS had selected to assess the quality of care provided to their active duty members and other beneficiaries. In addition, we interviewed the Chair of the Health Care Subcommittee of the Military Coalition, a group of 32 military, veterans, and uniformed services organizations. Although not representative, this allowed us to obtain the perspectives of beneficiaries on the MHS's quality measurement efforts.

To examine the extent to which DOD has established performance standards related to its core direct care measures and purchased care measures and corrective action requirements for providers that do not meet performance standards, we reviewed policies related to the MHS's oversight of provider performance on the measures on its Core and Purchased Care Dashboards. We also interviewed MHS officials and reviewed relevant MHS documents to determine whether the MHS sets specific performance standards for MTFs and civilian providers related to the quality measures on the Core and Purchased Care Dashboards. We also examined whether or to what extent MHS has established requirements for initiating corrective actions when providers do not meet those performance standards. The relevant documents we reviewed include the minutes of the MHS governance body meetings noted above; the MHS reports to Congress on direct and purchased care; documents related to the purchased care contracts; and reports that contractors submitted to the MHS for purchased care.[11] Additionally, in our review of the MHS governance body meeting

[11] U.S. Department on Defense, *Response to Section 730. Response to Section 713 of the National Defense Authorization Act for Fiscal Year 2016 (Public Law 114–92): Expansion of Evaluation of Effectiveness of the TRICARE Program to Include Information on Patient Safety, Quality of Care, and Access to Care at Military Treatment Facilities, May 22, 2017. Report to the Armed Services Committees on Pilot Program on Incorporation of Value-Based Health Care in Purchased Care Component of TRICARE Program, Section 701(h)(3) National Defense Authorization Act for Fiscal Year 2017 (Public Law 114-328), and Implementation Plan – Value-Based Incentives, Section 705(d) National Defense Authorization Act for Fiscal Year 2017 (Public Law 114-328), January 31, 2018.*

minutes, we examined MHS officials' decisions, their rationale, and any actions taken in response to the trends being monitored on the Core and Purchased Care Dashboard quality measures. We compared these MHS efforts to federal standards for internal control related to monitoring.[12]

We conducted this performance audit from June 2017 to September 2018 in accordance with generally accepted government auditing standards. Those standards require that we plan and perform the audit to obtain sufficient, appropriate evidence to provide a reasonable basis for our findings and conclusions based on our audit objectives. We believe that the evidence obtained provides a reasonable basis for our findings and conclusions based on our audit objectives.

BACKGROUND

Health Care Quality Measures

As we have previously reported in reviews of health care quality outside of the MHS, health care quality measures are standard, evidence-based metrics designed to assess the extent to which patients receive health care that increases the likelihood of desired health outcomes and are consistent with current professional knowledge.[13] These measures may be used to assess the quality of care in various settings, including hospitals and physician offices. Health care quality measures are intended to (1) inform providers about opportunities for potential improvements in their delivery of care, (2) encourage or incentivize providers to consistently provide high quality care, and (3) inform consumers about which providers are most

---

[12] Internal control is a process effected by an entity's oversight body, management, and other personnel that provides reasonable assurance that the objectives of an entity will be achieved. See GAO, *Standards for Internal Control in the Federal Government*, GAO-14-704G (Washington, D.C.: Sept. 2014).

[13] See GAO, *VA Health Care Quality: VA Should Improve the Information It Publicly Reports on the Quality of Care at Its Medical Facilities*, GAO-17-741, (Washington, D.C.: Sept. 2017) and GAO, *Health Care Quality: HHS Should Set Priorities and Comprehensively Plan Its Efforts to Better Align Health Quality Measures*, GAO-17-5, (Washington, D.C.: Oct. 2016).

likely to deliver high quality care. There are broad categories of clinical quality measures that address various aspects of quality of care. See Table 1 for a description of these broad categories of quality measures.

Table 1. Categories of Health Care Quality Measures

Measure category	Description	Examples
Process	Shows whether steps or processes of care that have been proven to benefit patients are followed correctly	The measures indicate whether an action was completed—such as writing a prescription, administering a drug, or having a conversation.
Outcome	Reports the actual results of care	The measures indicate a change in patient health status, such as lower blood pressure, for a patient who is hypertensive. They also include patient safety measures, which monitor the incidence of adverse events such as infections or complications.
Structural	Reflects the conditions in which providers care for patients.	The measures indicate staffing levels or the volume of procedures performed by a provider.
Patient experience	Records patients' perspectives on their care.	The measures reflect patient reports on their care, often obtained through surveys, such as patient responses to a question about whether their pain was always well controlled during a hospital stay.
Access	Assesses a patient's ability to obtain timely and appropriate care	The measures indicate the difficulty or length of time it takes for patients to receive health care services, such as an office visit with a physician.
Resource use	Assesses amount of resources expended to treat patients	The measures indicate the quantity of health care services used, such as the number of days in the hospital, or the average amount paid to treat certain conditions.

Source: GAO summary of information from the Agency for Health Care Research and Quality. | GAO-18-574.

The data used to calculate the results of health care quality measures can come from a number of different sources. Some measures often require detailed clinical information obtained from patient medical records, such as process measures that indicate whether timely and effective care was provided in a specific situation, for example, or whether stroke patients received clot-dissolving medication appropriately.

Other measures are designed to use information on patient demographics and diagnoses that can be obtained from more readily accessible sources, such as claims data or other administrative data that have already been collected for other purposes such as billing. In addition, patients can be asked directly, usually through surveys, to report on their experiences receiving care.

The MHS Structure and Administration of Direct and Purchased Care

The MHS is a complex organization in which responsibility for the delivery of health care is primarily shared among the military services—Army, Navy, and Air Force—and the Defense Health Agency (DHA).[14] The Army, Navy and Air Force medical commands report through their service chiefs to their respective military department Secretaries and then to the Secretary of Defense. DHA reports through the Office of the Assistant Secretary of Defense for Health Affairs and the Under Secretary of Defense for Personnel and Readiness to the Secretary of Defense. The Office of the Assistant Secretary of Defense for Health Affairs manages the Defense Health Program appropriation, which funds the medical and health care programs at the medical commands of the military services. As of fiscal year 2018, most of the MTFs, including military hospitals and clinics, were under the direction and control of the military services, which are responsible for staffing, training, and equipping those MTFs to meet mission requirements. DHA has responsibility for the managed care support contracts through which the MHS administers its purchased care, and DHA also administers

[14] The Navy is also responsible for delivery of health care services to the Marine Corps.

several MTFs in the vicinity of Washington, DC. Figure 1 depicts the MHS organizational structure.

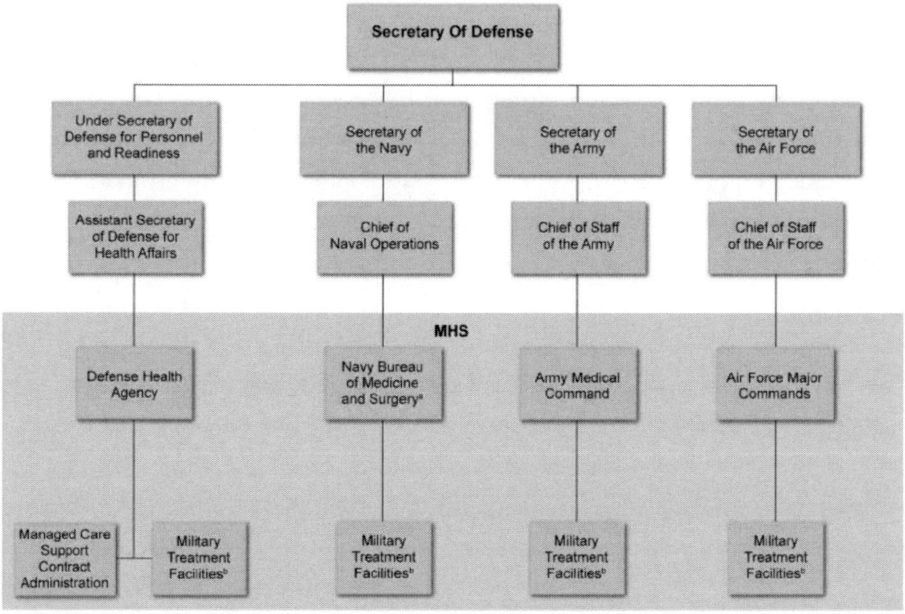

Source: Department of Defense. | GAO-18-574.

[a]The Navy is also responsible for delivery of health care services to the Marine Corps.

[b]Starting October 1, 2018, the Defense Health Agency will begin to assume responsibility for administering all military treatment facilities.

Figure 1. Organization of the Military Health System (MHS), as of Fiscal Year 2018.

Recently enacted changes will affect the administration of the MTFs in future years. Most notably, DOD will alter administration of the MTFs, shifting responsibility from the military services to DHA. Section 702 of the National Defense Authorization Act for Fiscal Year 2017 (NDAA 2017) directed DOD to give DHA responsibility for the administration of all MTFs, including budgetary matters, information technology, and health care administration and management.[15] In the conference report for NDAA 2017, Congress stated its intention that the creation of a single agency responsible for all MTFs would improve and sustain readiness, reduce costs, and

[15] Pub. L. No 114-328, § 702, 130 Stat. 2000, 2193 (2016).

increase efficiency. DOD has since prepared a series of implementation plans as it works to develop the specific policies and procedures to enable this change to take effect starting October 1, 2018. The most recent plan issued by DOD in June 2018 envisions a 3-year transition to be completed October 1, 2021.[16]

For purchased care, DOD contracts with civilian health care contractors to manage its civilian providers on a regional basis. The primary responsibilities of these managed care support contractors include the following:

- developing civilian provider networks, which include hospitals and clinicians;
- ensuring adequate access to health care;
- enrolling beneficiaries;
- referring and authorizing beneficiaries to receive health care;
- processing health care claims;
- educating providers and beneficiaries; and
- conducting utilization management and quality management programs.

There have been several generations of multi-year contracts since 1996. In July 2016, DOD awarded its fourth generation of managed care support contracts to two regional contractors, and on January 1, 2018, the MHS began health care delivery under these contracts.[17]

---

[16] Department of Defense, *Final Plan to Implement Section 1073c of Title 10, United States Code*, Report to the Armed Services Committees of the Senate and House of Representatives (June 30, 2018).

[17] A third contractor administers purchased care outside of the United States and the Uniformed Services Family Health Plan provides purchased care services under a separate capitated program in six designated locations.

Selection of Measures to Assess Quality of Direct and Purchased Care

According to our review of DOD documents, the MHS uses a structured process to select the measures on its dashboards that are used to assess the quality of direct and purchased care. Specifically, DOD documents state that the core direct care measures that are on the Core Dashboard are selected through the MHS's performance management system called Partnership for Improvement (P4I), which began in 2015.[18] The documents show that proposals for potential quality measures are developed by work groups that focus on different specialized areas, such as maternity care or mental health. These proposals are reviewed and approved by the Steering Committee for P4I, which develops the list of core quality measures for direct care. The Steering Committee then presents the list of core quality measures to a succession of governance bodies—each of which incorporates representation from the three military services plus DHA—for review and approval.[19] DOD documents indicate that the MHS repeats this process annually as it decides which quality measures to add, drop, or modify for the coming fiscal year from the Core Dashboard.[20]

The DOD documents we reviewed lay out a parallel process that the MHS follows to select which purchased care quality measures will be tracked in the Purchased Care Dashboard. A work group that specializes on

---

[18] The impetus for creating P4I was the finding of the 2014 comprehensive review of the MHS that MTFs delivered care of inconsistent quality. See Department of Defense, *Final Report to the Secretary of Defense, Military Health System Review* (August 2014). In response to the comprehensive review, the Secretary of Defense issued a memorandum that directed the MHS to develop a performance management system to manage and monitor the performance of all of the MTFs. Secretary of Defense, *Memorandum: Military Health System Action Plan for Access, Quality of Care, and Patient Safety*, Oct. 1, 2014.

[19] The governance bodies collaborate to develop various strategies to meet health policy directives and targets, and they oversee all of the MHS's health care policy decisions. They are, in order of increasing seniority, the Medical Operations Group, the Medical Deputies Action Group, and the Senior Military Medical Action Council.

[20] The MHS also selects from the full set of P4I measures a subset of measures on which to focus its quality improvement efforts. The MHS selected 13 such Process Improvement Priorities for fiscal year 2018.

purchased care issues with representation of DHA and the three military services develops the proposed list of quality measures for the Purchased Care Dashboard. This list is then reviewed and approved by the same succession of governance bodies that decide on the Core Dashboard measures.

Officials told us and DOD documents confirmed that the MHS and the purchased care contractors also track additional quality measures that are not included in the Core and Purchased Care Dashboards. For example, MHS clinicians who provide maternity care track a set of measures developed by the National Perinatal Information Center.[21] Similarly, a number of military hospitals report on surgical quality measures to the National Surgical Quality Improvement Program.[22] The MHS also conducts surveys of MHS beneficiaries from which it obtains data for patient experience measures for both direct and purchased care. Additionally, the MHS requires the managed care support contractors that administer the MHS's networks of civilian providers for purchased care to monitor several different sets of quality measures or indicators, many of which focus on patient safety. These include patient safety indicators, hospital acquired conditions, and serious reportable events.[23] They also analyze measures selected from Hospital Compare and the Healthcare Effectiveness Data and Information Set (HEDIS), some of which correspond to measures included in the Core and Purchased Care Dashboards.[24]

---

[21] The National Perinatal Information Center is a not-for-profit organization with expertise analyzing large data sets and developing comparative benchmarking quality measures, particularly for perinatal care. Perinatal care refers to both maternity care, which includes care provided to the mother before birth, care provided during labor and delivery, and care provided after birth; and neonatal care, which is care provided to the newborn.

[22] The National Surgical Quality Improvement Program uses measures that focus on complications or unintended events, such as morbidity, mortality, or readmission to the hospital, that occur within a 30-day period following hospitalization for different types of surgery. It is managed by the American College of Surgeons, a medical specialty society.

[23] Quality indicators, such as hospital acquired conditions and serious reportable events, typically identify individual instances of patient harm or inappropriate care.

[24] The National Committee for Quality Assurance created the HEDIS measure set to assess the performance of health plans.

The Hospital Compare and Core Quality Measures Collaborative Measure Sets Adopted by Medicare and Private Health Insurers

While health care systems in the United States can use a variety of measures to assess the quality of care, two of the most widely adopted sets of quality measures include the Hospital Compare measure set developed by Centers for Medicare & Medicaid Services (CMS) for inpatient care and the CQMC measure sets jointly developed by CMS and major private health insurers for outpatient care. Since 2005, CMS has collected results for individual hospitals on a specific list of health care quality measures that are posted on a website known as Hospital Compare. CMS does this to make comparable information on the quality of care provided by different hospitals publicly available. Hospital Compare currently covers more than 4,000 hospitals that participate in the Medicare program. These hospitals supply data to CMS for quality measures of inpatient and emergency department care.[25] These data reflect the care provided to all patients treated at these hospitals, not just those covered by Medicare. Each year CMS goes through a formal process, including receiving input from experts and stakeholders, to review and revise the mix of quality measures that these hospitals are expected to report. The purpose of this review, according to CMS, is to ensure that the set of measures reported on Hospital Compare provides meaningful information for quality improvement while reducing unnecessary administrative burden.[26]

Initiated in 2014, the CQMC is a multi-stakeholder voluntary effort focused on quality measure alignment that has developed eight sets of

---

[25] Hospitals report information for the inpatient Hospital Compare measures under the Medicare Hospital Inpatient Quality Reporting Program. Hospitals report information for emergency department care under the Medicare Hospital Outpatient Quality Reporting Program.

[26] Recently, the Department of Veterans Affairs also started supplying data to CMS for public reporting of quality measures of its hospitals.

measures for outpatient primary and specialty care, known as the CQMC measure sets.[27] In developing the measure sets, CMS and private health insurers negotiate sets of core measures on which they agree to focus on measuring care quality for certain conditions. Physician specialty societies, employer groups, consumer groups, and regional collaboratives also participate in the negotiations. The CQMC measure sets have been adopted by CMS for Medicare and by 15 major private health insurers for commercial health plans. Additionally, section 728 of the NDAA 2017 directs the MHS to use, to the extent appropriate, these quality measures to assess the quality of direct and purchased care.[28] CQMC documents show that the members of the CQMC intend to continually update these core measure sets as more meaningful measures are developed over time. CMS and the private health insurers plan to expand their application of these measures incrementally, as CMS conducts its annual reviews of Medicare's quality measures and the insurers update or renew their contracts with different providers.

THE MHS DOES NOT USE A COMMON SET OF QUALITY MEASURES FOR DIRECT AND PURCHASED CARE, AND THE MEASURES IT USES ASSESS A LIMITED RANGE OF QUALITY AREAS

The MHS does not use a common set of measures on its Core and Purchased Care Dashboards to assess the quality of care provided through direct and purchased care. In addition, for both direct and purchased care, the MHS uses measures on its dashboards that assess a more limited range of quality care areas and medical conditions as compared to the Hospital

[27] In February 2016, seven CQMC core measure sets were released that focused on primary care, cardiology, orthopedics, medical oncology, obstetrics and gynecology, gastroenterology, and HIV/hepatitis C. In July 2017, an eighth measure set focused on pediatrics was released.

[28] Pub. L. No. 114-328, § 728(a)(1), 130 Stat. 2000, 2233-2234 (2016).

Compare and CQMC measures adopted by Medicare and private health insurers.

The MHS Does Not Use a Common Set of Quality Measures for Direct and Purchased Care

Although the NDAA 2016 directed the MHS to align its quality measures for direct and purchased care, we found that as of March 31, 2018, the MHS used separate sets of measures on the Core and Purchased Care Dashboards to assess the quality of care delivered in direct and purchased care, respectively. To assess the quality of direct care, the MHS tracks 43 measures on its Core Dashboard, and to assess the quality of purchased care, the MHS tracks 18 measures on its Purchased Care Dashboard. The MHS tracks 8 measures that are the same for both dashboards, leaving 35 measures tracked only on the Core Dashboard for direct care and 10 measures tracked only on the Purchased Care Dashboard for purchased care (See Figure 2).

According to MHS officials, since launching the P4I performance management system in 2015, the MHS has focused on making systematic improvements in the quality of care across the MTFs in direct care. As a result, the 43 measures they have chosen for the Core Dashboard reflect their priorities for quality improvement within direct care only. In the case of purchased care, MHS officials stated that requiring civilian providers to report on the same 43 measures that are used on the Core Dashboard for direct care would add burden, and the MHS had concerns that this would make civilian providers less likely to participate in purchased care.[29] Instead, the MHS tracks 18 measures on the Purchased Care Dashboard that rely on information sources other than provider reporting, such as claims that the providers submit in the normal course of receiving payment for their services

---

[29] Recent research indicates that the overall burden placed on U.S. health care providers by multiple quality reporting programs is substantial and increasing, leading many providers to be skeptical about the value of reporting larger numbers of quality measures. See, for example, L.P. Casalino, et al., "U.S. Physician Practices Spend More Than $15.4 Billion Annually to Report Quality Measures," *Health Affairs*, 35:3 (2016) 401-406.

and surveys that the MHS conducts of its beneficiaries.[30] MHS officials explained that they try to minimize the reporting burden for purchased care providers because for most of these civilian providers, eligible MHS beneficiaries represent only a small proportion of their patient population.

We also found that for direct care, the MHS uses its quality measures on the Core Dashboard to assess the quality of care delivered to beneficiaries served by individual MTFs, such as hospitals or clinics. However, for purchased care, the MHS uses its quality measures on the Purchased Care Dashboard to assess the quality of care delivered to the beneficiary population served by each contractor's network as a whole– not the quality of care delivered by individual civilian hospitals, clinicians, or other providers in the network. Specifically:

- In direct care, the MHS uses the 43 measures on the Core Dashboard to track the quality of care delivered by individual MTFs. For example, on a measure of central line-associated bloodstream infections, the MHS tracks the incidence of such infections by individual MTF and by military service (i.e., the incidence of such infections in Army, Navy and Air Force MTFs).
- In contrast, in purchased care, the MHS assesses information on the 18 measures on the Purchased Care Dashboard for all beneficiaries in each of the networks administered by the two managed care support contractors. For example, on a measure of the percentage of beneficiaries with diabetes who have their hemoglobin level tested annually, the MHS calculates an overall rate of hemoglobin testing across all the diabetic patients that receive care in each contractor's network.

The beneficiary population-level reporting on quality measures on the Purchased Care Dashboard reflects the nature of the MHS's relationship

---

[30] For example, the MHS assesses outpatient care from purchased care providers using several HEDIS measures that are designed to determine if certain processes that represent good quality of care, such as testing the hemoglobin levels of diabetic patients annually, were or were not provided, based on the claims that providers submit for payment.

with its managed care support contractors for purchased care. Under the terms of the contracts that the MHS has negotiated with the contractors that administer the networks of civilian providers to care for eligible beneficiaries, the contractors bear responsibility for ensuring the quality of care delivered by those providers. While the MHS requires the managed care support contractors to monitor different sets of quality measures or indicators, such as patient safety indicators, hospital acquired conditions, and serious reportable events to identify possible cases of individual patient harm and determine appropriate interventions, the contractors report this information in annual reports to the MHS for their network as a whole, as opposed to reporting on individual providers.

Because the MHS largely uses separate measures for direct and purchased care on its dashboards and tracks the quality of care delivered by civilian providers in purchased care in the aggregate rather than individually, the MHS lacks the information it needs to make comparable assessments of the quality of care delivered across the MHS as a whole.

This, in turn, limits the MHS's ability to ensure it has the information needed to determine whether it is achieving the department's overall strategic goals of providing high quality care across the MHS as a whole and ensuring that beneficiaries receive a consistent level of high quality care regardless of whether that care is delivered in direct or purchased care. Moreover, using a different set of quality of measures on the dashboards for direct and purchased care is inconsistent with section 730 of the NDAA 2016, which directs the MHS to align its measures for direct and purchased care so it can reduce performance variation across the MHS.

MHS officials acknowledge in principle the value of using aligned measures to assess quality of care in direct and purchased care, but the officials cited a range of factors that pose challenges to achieving this objective, such as the large number of civilian providers and the lack of common health information technology systems.

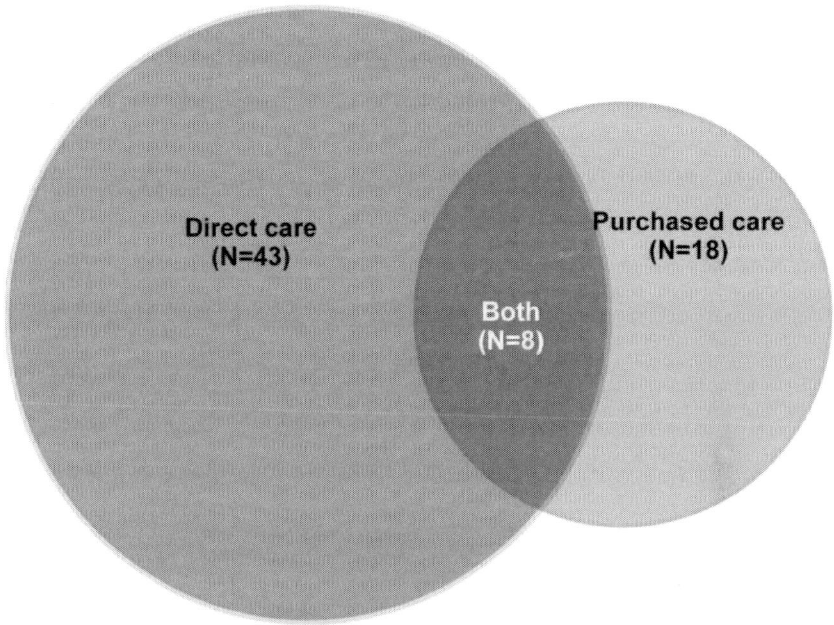

Source: GAO analysis of DOD data. | GAO-18-574.

Notes: Direct care refers to the care beneficiaries receive in the MHS's military treatment facilities. The quality measures for direct care are those that the MHS includes on its Core Dashboard. Purchased care refers to the care beneficiaries receive in civilian hospitals and by civilian clinicians that participate in health plans sponsored by the Department of Defense (DOD). The quality measures for purchased care are those that the MHS has selected to track on a separate Purchased Care dashboard. The MHS reported to the Congress that the measures on the Core and Purchased Care dashboards are the key measures that the Department of Defense's senior health care leadership uses to track progress in achieving overall strategic goals to provide high quality care.

Figure 2. Number of Core and Purchased Care Dashboard Quality Measures for Direct and Purchased Care in the Military Health System (MHS), as of March 31, 2018.

Based on our review, we found that one way the MHS could have a common set of quality measures for both direct and purchased care, without increasing the reporting burden on civilian providers, would be to use, as appropriate, Hospital Compare and CQMC quality measures. Notably, the MHS states on its website that almost all of the civilian hospitals that are in the contractors' networks for purchased care already report information on the measures posted on the Hospital Compare website. As a result, there potentially would be no additional burden for these purchased care providers to report information on the Hospital Compare quality measures. Similarly, major health plans report that they have begun implementing the CQMC measure sets in their contracts with physicians, meaning that physicians participating in those plans already report information on CQMC outpatient quality measures. To the extent that those physicians are also in the MHS contractors' networks for purchased care, the information the physicians report on the CQMC measures could be used by the MHS.[31]

We found the MHS is already using some Hospital Compare and CQMC measures for inpatient and outpatient care. There are a total of 76 measures that Medicare and private health insurers report to Hospital Compare and a total of 60 CQMC outpatient measures. Besides the measures used in the Core and Purchased Care Dashboards, MHS also collects 24 of 76 Hospital Compare measures and 10 of the 60 CQMC outpatient measures. For the most part, these measures are not part of the direct and purchased care dashboards that MHS leadership uses to assess the performance of direct and purchased care. Furthermore, MHS officials told us that they have no specific plans to increase the number of measures that the MHS uses from Hospital Compare for inpatient care delivered in its hospitals. In the case of outpatient care, our review of DOD documents shows that the MHS plans on expanding reporting to only 5 more CQMC quality measures, in large part to minimize its reporting burden.[32]

---

[31] Section 728 of the NDAA 2017 directs the MHS to use to the extent appropriate CQMC quality measures to assess the quality of direct and purchased care. Pub. L. No. 114-328, § 728(a)(1), 130 Stat. 2000, 2233-2234 (2016).

[32] For example, the MHS work group that recommended the MHS's approach for implementing Section 728 rejected adoption of CQMC measures that would require abstraction of clinical data from patient medical records, because, according to the group, such abstraction was expensive and time consuming.

The MHS Uses Quality Measures that Assess a Limited Range of Quality Care Areas and Medical Conditions Compared to Measures Adopted by Medicare and Private Health Insurers

We found that the measures the MHS uses on its Core and Purchased Care Dashboards to assess the quality of direct and purchased care address only a limited range of quality areas and medical conditions when compared with the Hospital Compare and CQMC measure sets that are adopted by Medicare and private health insurers. According to the National Quality Forum, which plays a central role in developing and annually reassessing the Hospital Compare measure set and also was consulted in the development of the CQMC measure sets, the measures used to assess quality of care should comprise an appropriate mix of recognized measure types, including outcome measures, process measures, experience of care measures, and cost and structure measures.[33] These measures should cover a broad enough range of measure types and medical conditions so that they provide an accurate overall assessment of the quality of care patients receive.

Based on our analysis, Table 2 below shows the limited range of measures on the Core and Purchased Care dashboards used by the MHS to assess inpatient care, as compared to the range of inpatient measures that Medicare hospitals report for Hospital Compare. In general, each of the five types of measures shown in the table below addresses different aspects of health care quality in hospital settings.

For direct care, the MHS uses no more than one measure on its Core Dashboard for all of these five measure types except for "Outcome" measures; for purchased care, the MHS does not use any inpatient care measures on its Purchased Care Dashboard.

---

[33] [3]National Quality Forum, "NQF Report on 2017 Activities to Congress and the Secretary of the Department of Health and Human Services," (Washington, DC: March 1, 2018), 80- 81. The National Quality Forum is a nonprofit organization that serves as the lead entity in the United States for endorsing health care quality measures and determining which measures should be recognized as national standards.

Table 2. Inpatient Quality Measures Used by the Military Health System (MHS) on Its Core and Purchased Care Dashboards as Compared with Measures on Hospital Compare, as of March 31, 2018

n/a	Number of inpatient measures		
Measure type[a]	MHS's Core Dashboard for direct care[b]	MHS's Purchased Care Dashboard for purchased care[c]	Medicare hospitals report to Hospital Compare[d]
Process (timely & effective care)	1	0	20
Outcome	9	0	26
Structural	0	0	8
Patient experience	1	0	11
Resource use	1	0	11
Total	12	0	76

Source: GAO analysis of information from the MHS and the Centers for Medicare & Medicaid Services | GAO-18-574.

[a]Measures are categorized according to the Agency for Healthcare Research and Quality's Measure Domain Framework.

[b]Direct care refers to the care beneficiaries receive in the MHS's military treatment facilities. The MHS reported to the Congress that the measures on the Core Dashboard are the key measures that the Department of Defense's (DOD) senior health care leadership uses to track progress in achieving overall strategic goals to provide high quality care.

[c]Purchased care refers to the care beneficiaries receive in civilian hospitals and by civilian clinicians that participate in DOD-sponsored health plans. The MHS reported to the Congress that the measures on the Purchased Care Dashboard are the key measures that the Department of Defense's senior health care leadership uses to track progress in achieving overall strategic goals to provide high quality care.

[d]The Centers for Medicare & Medicaid Services' Hospital Compare website provides consumers with information on the quality of care at over 4,000 hospitals that participate in Medicare.

Similarly, based on our analysis, Table 3 below shows the limited range of measures on the Core and Purchased Care Dashboards used by the MHS to assess outpatient care, as compared to the range of outpatient measures that are part of the CQMC measure sets adopted by Medicare and private health insurers. The MHS uses measures on its dashboards that assess fewer clinical focus areas and medical conditions as compared with those measures included in the CQMC measure sets.[34] As with hospital care, the difference is greatest with respect to purchased care.

The limitations we found in the quality measures used by the MHS—the relatively narrow range of measures as well as the relatively few measures used across direct and purchased care—reflect the MHS's priorities in selecting quality measures. In short, the MHS focuses on the value and impact of implementing individual measures, but does not prioritize aligning the measures used across direct and purchased care or expanding the range of medical conditions and quality areas covered in the aggregate by the measures. The MHS's annual assessment of quality measures focuses only the Core Dashboard measures. For each Core Dashboard measure for which a change is under consideration—such as dropping, modifying, or adding another quality measure to the Core Dashboard—MHS officials apply a standard set of criteria involving both the feasibility of collecting the data needed for that measure and the utility of that measure for addressing a strategic priority or promoting performance improvement.[35] When asked about the potential value of increasing the number of Hospital Compare measures, MHS officials said they need to make a value-based determination of whether the benefits of obtaining results for any given Hospital Compare measure justified the costs of collecting and transmitting the data required for that measure. In discussions about potential measures for the Purchased Care Dashboard, MHS officials also focused on the characteristics of specific measures being considered for inclusion in the dashboard.

[34] For example, measures in the clinical focus area of cardiology would address such medical conditions as heart failure, hypertension, and recuperation from a heart attack. Measures in the area of medical oncology would address therapies provided for different types of cancer, such as breast cancer or colorectal cancer.

[35] The initial set of measures for the Purchased Care Dashboard was formally adopted by the MHS in September 2017. The MHS has announced that it expects to add and remove measures from the Dashboard sometime in the future.

Table 3. Outpatient Quality Measures Used by the Military Health System (MHS) on Its Core and Purchased Care Dashboards as Compared with Measures Included in the Core Quality Measures Collaborative (CQMC) Measure Sets, as of March 31, 2018

	Number of inpatient measures		
Clinical focus areas of measures	**MHS's Core Dashboard for direct care[a]**	**MHS's Purchased Care Dashboard for purchased care[b]**	**Included in the CQMC measure sets[c]**
Behavioral health	1	1	0
Cardiovascular	0	0	8
Dental	0	1	0
Gastroenterology	0	0	8
HIV/Hepatitis C	0	0	8
Medical oncology	0	0	12
Obstetrics and gynecology	2	0	6
Orthopedic	0	0	1
Pediatric	2	3	5
Primary care	12	4	19
Total[d]	15	9	60

Source: GAO analysis of information from the MHS and the Centers for Medicare & Medicaid Services | GAO-18-574.

[a]Direct care refers to the care beneficiaries receive in the MHS's military treatment facilities. The MHS reported to the Congress that the measures on the Core Dashboard are the key measures that the Department of Defense's (DOD) senior health care leadership uses to track progress in achieving overall strategic goals to provide high quality care.

[b]Purchased care refers to the care beneficiaries receive in civilian hospitals and by civilian clinicians that participate in DOD-sponsored health plans. The MHS reported to the Congress that the measures on the Purchased Care Dashboard are the key measures that the Department of Defense's senior health care leadership uses to track progress in achieving overall strategic goals to provide high quality care.

[c]The Core Quality Measure Collaborative is a multi-stakeholder voluntary effort on quality measure alignment that includes representatives of the Centers for Medicare & Medicaid Services, major private health insurers, and medical specialty societies that has led to the development of eight sets of measures for outpatient care. Each of the eight CQMC measure sets is focused on a specific clinical focus area.

[d]The total may be less than the sum of the rows above because specific measures were only counted once even if they were used in measure sets for multiple clinical focus areas.

Because the MHS does not prioritize expanding the range of medical conditions and quality areas covered by common measures across direct and purchased care, the measures the MHS uses provide DOD's senior health care leadership with an incomplete picture of the quality of care across the MHS. As we have noted, the MHS has reported to the Congress that its DOD health care leaders rely on the Core and Purchased Care Dashboard measures to establish accountability throughout the MHS and identify areas where quality improvement is needed. However, the current approach may not lead to the selection of quality measures for the two dashboards that would enable MHS officials to identify the most critical quality of care issues in the MHS. The lack of that information, in turn, limits the ability of DOD's senior health care leadership to target their performance improvement efforts most effectively in support of DOD's overall strategic goals of providing high quality care across the MHS as a whole.

THE MHS HAS ESTABLISHED PERFORMANCE STANDARDS AND RELATED CORRECTIVE ACTION REQUIREMENTS FOR INDIVIDUAL PROVIDERS IN DIRECT CARE BUT NOT IN PURCHASED CARE

The MHS has established performance standards in direct care related to the Core Dashboard measures and has corrective action requirements for MTFs that do not meet the standards. However, the MHS has not established performance standards related to the Purchased Care Dashboard measures for individual civilian providers in purchased care and therefore does not have related corrective action requirements for these providers.

The MHS Has Established Direct Care Performance Standards and Related Corrective Action Requirements for Military Treatment Facilities

As part of its P4I performance management system for direct care, the MHS has established specific performance standards that each MTF must meet in delivering quality care to MHS beneficiaries. These standards—

some of which are under development—specify a minimum level of performance that each MTF should achieve related to the Core Dashboard quality measures tracked in direct care.[36] For example, in the case of the HEDIS All Cause Readmission measure on the Core Dashboard, the MHS's performance standard is that MTFs should have a rate of unplanned acute readmissions within 30 days of an initial hospital admission that is as good as or better than the national 75th percentile.[37] This performance standard is based on the readmission rates that the National Committee for Quality Assurance, the lead entity for that measure, has observed across U.S. hospitals.

During regularly recurring governance meetings throughout the year, MHS governance bodies review how MTFs have performed relative to the performance standards for the Core Dashboard measures.[38] Our review found that during these meetings, the governance bodies generally do not examine the circumstances of MTFs that do not perform well on the performance standards related to the Core Dashboard measures. Consequently, DOD's senior health care leadership within the governance bodies may receive limited information on the challenges faced by low-performing individual MTFs. However, during these meetings, officials from the military services and DHA highlight MTFs that are performing well

---

[36] The MHS has established performance standards related to 37 of the 43 quality measures it tracks on the Core Dashboard for direct care. For the remaining 6 measures, performance standards were under development as of March 31, 2018. The performance standards are the same for all MTFs across the different military services. The MHS establishes its performance standards through the same process that it uses for selecting its Core Dashboard measures for direct care. The P4I Steering Committee proposes performance standards, along with associated rationales, to the governance bodies for review and approval. The governance bodies then have the opportunity to discuss the specific values of the proposed thresholds, asking questions or voicing concerns about the particular methodology underpinning a measure.

[37] The National Committee for Quality Assurance benchmarks the performance of the plans that report on the HEDIS measures in terms of percentiles. Performance at the 75th percentile represents the level that is as good or better than that reported by 75 percent of health plans submitting data for this measure.

[38] These governance meetings take place weekly, monthly, or quarterly, depending on the governance body.

on the established performance standards, and the officials share best practices and specific strategies used to achieve high performance.[39]

We also found that in direct care, the MHS requires MTFs that do not meet the MHS's performance standards related to its Core Dashboard measures to take corrective actions to improve the quality of care they deliver. The military services—Army, Navy and Air Force—and DHA have been responsible for implementing this requirement. For example, Navy officials explained that they periodically review information collected on the MHS's Core Dashboard quality measures to analyze areas where MTFs do not meet established performance standards tied to these measures and to oversee MTFs' efforts to correct these deficiencies.[40] Officials told us that each of the services exercises its discretion to independently develop and implement the corrective actions that the service determines best address the performance issues identified through the use of the MHS's quality measures.[41] For example, to help reduce the number of Central Line-Associated Bloodstream Infections (CLABSI), the Army began financially awarding MTFs that performed well on the CLABSI measure, whereas the Air Force developed a toolkit to help providers prevent CLABSI.

As the MHS moves to transfer administration of the MTFs from the individual military services to DHA as directed by section 702 of the NDAA 2017, the approach for assessing performance and implementing corrective actions is likely to change. The MHS's recently issued implementation plan as of June 2018 outlines some alterations to the current performance assessment process.[42] Specifically, MTFs will create and submit a performance plan that will be reviewed and approved by DHA. DHA will

---

[39] The emphasis on high performance reflects the MHS's effort, highlighted in the MHS 2014 Review and other MHS documents, to establish an organizational culture that promotes open discussion of quality and safety issues without fear of blame or reprisal.

[40] Navy officials told us and our review of Navy documents shows that the Navy monitors its MTFs' performance on the Core Dashboard measures as well as on quality measures that the Navy independently decided to track. For example, the Navy monitors Navy enrollment per full time employee, no show rates, and the percentage of patients asked to call back for an appointment.

[41] For the MTFs that DHA administers, DHA also uses its discretion to determine corrective actions to address quality performance issues.

[42] Department of Defense, *Final Plan to Implement Section 1073c of Title 10, United States Code*, Report to the Armed Services Committees of the Senate and House of Representatives (June 30, 2018).

host monthly review sessions with MTFs to track performance on the plan. MTFs will be evaluated using a set of measures aligned to the Quadruple Aim that will include many but not all of the Core Dashboard measures.

The MHS Has Not Established Performance Standards and Related Corrective Action Requirements for Individual Civilian Providers in Purchased Care

The MHS has not established performance standards related to the 18 Purchased Care Dashboard measures for individual civilian hospitals, clinicians, or other providers in purchased care. Instead, the MHS has established performance standards related to the 18 Purchased Care Dashboard measures that MHS officials use to track the performance of each of the two managed care support contractors.[43] According to MHS officials, the MHS does not require the contractors to ensure that each individual hospital, physician, or other provider in these networks meets the performance standards related to the Purchased Care Dashboard measures. For example, in the case of a measure on the use of imaging for low back pain, the MHS has set a performance standard for each managed care support contractor, one that aims at avoiding excessive imaging across the beneficiary population in the contractor's network. However, officials told us that the information that the MHS collects on the measure—the number of beneficiaries in each of the contractors' networks who receive imaging services for low back pain—does not indicate the extent to which each individual civilian provider in the contractor networks meets or fails to meet the performance standard. Thus, the information the MHS obtains on the quality measure and its related performance standard does not identify which hospitals, clinicians, or other providers need to improve their performance in order for all beneficiaries to receive the expected level of care quality that the performance standard represents.

---

[43] As we have noted, the MHS assigns broad responsibility to the managed care support contractors to help ensure the quality of care provided by their individual network providers.

Because the MHS has not established performance standards related to the Purchased Care dashboard measures for individual civilian hospitals, clinicians, or other providers in purchased care, there are no related requirements for corrective action. Instead, the MHS requires its managed care support contractors to undertake other activities to promote improved quality of care across civilian providers in their networks. These include investigations of quality issues, focused reviews, analyses of Hospital Compare data, and value-based purchasing pilots, as discussed further below. However, our review found that these efforts are not applied comprehensively across all individual purchased care providers.

Investigations of Quality Issues

One approach the MHS uses to promote improved quality of care across purchased care providers is to direct its managed care support contractors to investigate whether individual beneficiaries have experienced what the MHS refers to as a quality issue. Potential quality issues are defined by the MHS as any instance when there are indications that a purchased care provider has deviated from what the managed care support contractors deem acceptable standards of professional practice. The contractors can identify these potential quality issues through beneficiary complaints; analyses of patient safety indicators, hospital acquired conditions, and serious reportable events; or by the MHS or contractor staff. Once potential quality issues are identified, they are investigated by a clinician, who reviews the patient's complete medical record. Based on the clinician's review of the patient's medical records, the clinician verifies whether or not a quality issue has occurred and, if so, assigns the quality issue a severity level.[44] To address the quality issue, the managed care support contractors may take a range of steps, including educating the provider, monitoring the provider, notifying the appropriate state or federal bodies, and removing the provider from the MHS's purchased care provider network. In practice, however, MHS

---

[44] The severity of the quality levels are rated 1-4 or are classified sentinel events. Severity level 1 represents a quality issue with minimal potential for significant adverse effects on the patient, whereas severity level 4 represents a quality issue with the most severe adverse effect and warrants exhaustive review. A sentinel event is a quality issue that results in death, permanent harm, severe temporary harm, or intervention required to sustain life.

officials said and documents we reviewed show that providers are rarely removed from the network. For example, MHS officials reported that one contractor estimated that one provider was removed from its network over quality issues every 1 to 2 years.

Focused Reviews

Another way the MHS uses its managed care support contractors to promote improved quality of care across purchased care providers is through focused reviews. During these reviews, the managed care support contractors review the medical records for a selected patient population to determine the extent to which a specified quality concern is a widespread problem. For example, in 2015 one contractor reviewed the medical records of 96 beneficiaries to determine the frequency of obstetric trauma, an injury related to vaginal deliveries. If a focused review determines that there is a widespread quality problem, the contractor may implement a quality improvement initiative designed to prompt all of its network providers to address that concern, as opposed to targeting specific providers.

Analyses of Hospital Compare Data

The MHS also requires the contractors to conduct an annual examination of the performance of hospitals in their networks on the different quality measures reported on Medicare's Hospital Compare. However, the managed care support contractors have considerable flexibility in deciding how to structure these analyses and how to follow-up on results. Consequently, the two managed care support contractors have adopted different analytical approaches to define and identify hospitals with relatively low performance.[45] For example, the managed care support contractors chose to examine different quality measures and use different criteria to identify hospitals with relatively low performance. In their most recent annual reports issued during 2017, both managed care support contractors indicated that they were considering contacting the lower performing hospitals to

---

[45] The Hospital Compare analyses conducted by the managed care support contractors identify hospitals that perform less well than other hospitals in their networks, but the analyses do not indicate whether hospitals have met a set performance standard.

prompt remedial action, but because no action had yet occurred, the reports leave open what steps were ultimately taken and how these hospitals responded. Nonetheless, these activities suggest that the managed care support contractors have the ability to use Hospital Compare to analyze and address individual provider performance on a standard set of quality measures. However, the MHS has not specified how this process should proceed, leaving it to the managed care support contractors to decide what and how much they will do in conducting these analyses of individual hospitals.

Value-Based Purchasing Pilots

The MHS has recently begun to test different approaches to incentivize purchased care providers to deliver high quality care through several value-based purchasing pilots.[46] For example, in February 2018 the MHS launched a maternity care pilot that pays providers more for better performance on specified quality measures. The pilot also implements a 'steerage model' approach that identifies higher performing providers in directories provided to patients by indicating providers as "Gold Stork" or "Silver Stork." These pilots may provide the MHS another way to influence the quality of care provided by certain subsets of its purchased care providers. MHS officials stated that although DOD has not arrived at specific goals, it plans to expand these pilots to cover around 20 to 25 percent of its purchased care services by 2020. The use of performance standards and corrective action requirements for individual hospitals, clinicians, or other providers who serve MHS beneficiaries is consistent with federal internal control standards for monitoring, which state that management should establish monitoring activities, evaluate the results, and remediate any deficiencies.[47] While the MHS has established performance standards related to its Core Dashboard measures in direct care and has corrective action requirements for MTFs that do not meet those standards, it has not done so for individual civilian

---

[46] NDAA 2017 directed the Secretary to carry out pilot programs to demonstrate and assess the feasibility of incorporating a value-based health care methodology into purchased care no later than January 1, 2018. NDAA 2017, Pub. L. No. 114-328, § 701(h), 130 Stat. 2000, 2188 (2016).

[47] See GAO-14-704G.

hospitals, clinicians, or other providers in purchased care related to its Purchased Care Dashboard measures. Additionally, if the MHS aligned quality measures on the Core and Purchased Care Dashboards at the provider level, the MHS could require its managed care support contractors to monitor the performance of individual civilian providers relative to set performance standards comparable to the ones that the MHS has established for MTFs. This approach would allow the MHS to determine the extent of performance variability, both among individual civilian providers and across MTFs and individual civilian providers. By not establishing consistent performance standards at the provider-level for direct and purchased care and requiring corrective action requirements to ensure that these standards are met by providers in both direct and purchased care, the MHS is limited in its ability to address variation in the quality of care delivered. This further limits the MHS's ability to ensure that it is achieving the department's overall strategic goals of providing high quality care across the MHS as whole and ensuring that beneficiaries receive a consistent level of high quality care regardless of whether that care is delivered in direct or purchased care.

CONCLUSION

Congress directed DOD to reduce variation in the quality of care beneficiaries receive through the MHS. DOD has taken important steps towards this goal by identifying a set of core measures that DOD senior health care leadership use to assess quality of care in direct care and another set of measures that they use to assess quality in purchased care. DOD health care leaders rely on these measures on their Core and Purchased Care Dashboards to establish accountability throughout the MHS and identify areas where quality improvement is needed. However, with few exceptions, the MHS uses different measures on its Core and Purchased Care Dashboards to assess the quality of direct and purchased care, making it difficult to determine the extent to which it is ensuring consistent quality across the MHS as a whole. Furthermore, for both direct and purchased care, the MHS uses measures on its dashboards that assess a limited range of quality areas and medical conditions when compared to the widely used quality measure sets adopted by Medicare and private insurers. Without using a broader range of available quality measures available—measures that many purchased care providers already report to CMS and private health insurers—DOD is missing an opportunity to better target the most critical quality of care issues in the MHS. The limitations we identified in the MHS's Core and Purchased Care Dashboard quality measures reflect the fact that in its annual measure selection process, the MHS does not prioritize aligning the quality measures across direct and purchased care and expanding the range of measures it uses across the two systems of care.

Finally, our review shows that while DOD has established performance standards for the core measures in direct care and corrective action requirements for MTFs that do not meet these standards, DOD has not done so for individual purchased care providers. Notably, DOD does not set clear expectations that individual purchased care providers should meet the performance standards related to the quality measures on the Purchased Care Dashboard. Performance standards and related corrective action requirements are critical for holding both MTFs and individual civilian providers accountable for providing quality care. Without consistent standards and related corrective action requirements across the MHS, DOD is limited in its ability to ensure that beneficiaries consistently receive high quality care, regardless of whether they receive that care in the direct or purchased care systems.

RECOMMENDATIONS FOR EXECUTIVE ACTION

We are making two recommendations to the Assistant Secretary of Defense for Health Affairs.

As MHS governing bodies conduct their recurring reviews of quality measures selected for MHS's Core Dashboard and Purchased Care Dashboards, the Assistant Secretary of Defense for Health Affairs should direct those bodies to prioritize, as appropriate, the selection of measures that apply to both direct and purchased care at the provider level and that expand the range of quality measure types and medical conditions that are assessed. (Recommendation 1)

The Assistant Secretary of Defense for Health Affairs should establish, as appropriate, performance standards related to the Purchased Care Dashboard measures that are consistent with the MHS's performance standards for direct care; ensure they are applied to individual purchased care providers; and take steps, such as amending its managed care support contracts, if necessary, to require corrective actions to be taken when providers do not meet those standards. (Recommendation 2)

AGENCY COMMENTS AND OUR EVALUATION

We provided a draft of this chapter to DOD for review, and DOD provided written comments, which are reprinted in appendix I. In its written comments, DOD concurred with both of our recommendations. With regards to the first recommendation, DOD stated that it plans to enhance the process for selecting quality measures that apply to both direct and purchased care; optimize use of data on Hospital Compare to expand the types and medical conditions evaluated; augment their governance reporting structure so that senior leadership can review quality measures included on the Core Dashboard and Purchased Care Dashboard; and implement the CQMC measure sets for outpatient care. Additionally, DOD stated that it has efforts underway to create a library of all quality measures used across direct and purchased care.

With regards to the second recommendation, DOD acknowledged the need to strengthen accountability for meeting performance standards that apply to both direct and purchased care providers. It also agreed that measures of individual provider performance in purchased care should be augmented and consistent with measures in direct care, where possible. DOD noted, however, that because it works through managed care support contractors for purchased care, it can hold the contractors accountable for meeting performance standards but cannot currently take action against individual providers based solely on performance. Instead, DOD stated that rather than taking a corrective action approach, it plans to expand its value-based purchasing efforts and incentivize providers that meet and exceed certain quality standards. This raises concerns, as DOD's current plans to expand its value-based purchasing efforts would only be applicable for between 20 and 25 percent of the services MHS beneficiaries receive from purchased care providers by 2020, as we noted in our report. Without having all providers managed consistently and subject to prompt remediation of deficiencies, DOD is missing an opportunity to improve the quality of purchased care, and it increases the risk that not all beneficiaries will receive a consistent level of high quality care across the MHS. Acknowledging DOD's comment that it cannot currently take action against individual providers based solely on performance, we have modified our recommendation to clarify that DOD should take the steps it determines are necessary, such as amending its managed care support contracts, to institute corrective action requirements for purchased care providers.

Sharon M. Silas
Acting Director,
Health Care

APPENDIX I: COMMENTS FROM THE DEPARTMENT OF DEFENSE

Aug 31 2018
Ms. Sharon Silas
Acting Director, Health Care
U.S. Government Accountability Office
441 G Street, NW
Washington, DC 20548

Dear Ms. Silas:

The enclosed is the Department of Defense (DoD) response to the Government Accountability Office (GAO) Draft Report GAO-18-574, “Expanded Use of Quality Measures Could Enhance Oversight of Provider Performance.”

Sincerely,

Tom McCaffery

Principal Deputy Assistant Secretary of Defense for Health Affairs Enclosure:

Government Accountability Office (GAO)

Draft Report Dated July 27, 2018

GAO-18-574 (GAO Code 102107)

“Defense Health Care: Expanded Use of Quality Measures Could Enhance Oversight of Provider Performance”

Department of Defense Comments to the Gao Recommendation

Recommendation 1: The GAO recommendation for the Assistant Secretary of Defense for Health Affairs (ASD(HA)) as follows: As Military Health System (MHS) governing bodies conduct their recurring reviews of quality measures selected for MHS’s Core Dashboard and Purchased Care Dashboards, the ASD(HA) should direct those bodies to prioritize, as appropriate, the selection of measures that apply to both direct and purchased care at the provider level and that expand the range of quality measure types and medical conditions that are assessed. (Recommendation 1)

Department of Defense (DoD) Response: The Department concurs with the recommendation.

The Defense Health Agency (DHA) has recently developed a High Reliability Organization Operating Model, leveraging subject matter expertise in Clinical Communities to establish overarching care pathways for patient experience that will eliminate harm, reduce unwarranted variation, improve patient outcomes and increase value for all stakeholders, regardless of the environment the patient used to access the MHS for an episode of care (direct, purchased, deployed). With the Readiness mission as the priority, Clinical Communities (with representation from DHA Purchased Care) are working to establish standards for patient outcomes and improvements to processes to achieve those outcomes. Though data capture analysis of clinical process improvement is anticipated to be more streamlined for direct care through configuration of DoD's new Electronic Medical Record, Purchased Care supports this work investigating alternative means to show alignment with strategic and clinical analysis of patient care priorities. The DHA is continuously improving the means by which care pathways are aligned and resourced per strategic guidance in the MHS Quadruple Aim Performance Plan. Accordingly, this will improve the review process of measures that apply to both direct and Purchased Care at the provider level, with a specific focus on expanding the range of quality measure types and medical conditions that are assessed by:

1) Enhancing process for selection of measures reported to MHS Leadership, to include prioritization of measures by applicability to both direct and Purchased Care; availability of provider level data; quality measure types; and medical condition focus.
2) Optimizing the National Hospital Quality Measures (NHQM) data available on Hospital Compare to expand the types and medical conditions that are evaluated through quality measures for both direct and Purchased Care.
3) Augmenting the governance reporting structure to allow for senior leadership to review additional quality measures to those included on the MHS's Core and Purchased Care Dashboards.
4) Collaborating with Centers for Medicare and Medicaid (CMS) and National Quality Forum (NQF) in the development phase of implementing Core Quality Measures Collaborative (CQMC) measure sets.

Quality measures currently reported on MHS's Core and Purchased Care Dashboards represent only a subset of data collected to assess the quality of care delivered in the MHS. The Purchased Care Dashboard represents only one method of communicating quality performance to leadership. A limited number of measures on the Purchased Care Dashboard is intentional to be manageable in scope. Additionally, several measures on the Core Dashboard, such as the force readiness and medical skills readiness measures, are not applicable to individual Purchased Care providers.

Current efforts are underway to create a library of all clinical measures used by DHA (to include measures on the Dashboards) for knowledge management - a means to provide reference on what measure was used, and why it was developed (i.e., what strategic question was it answering or supporting). Analysis of these measures and their applicability to both direct and purchased care can support strategic guidance and future selection of measures for the Core and Purchased Care Dashboards.

In addition to the above, measures from the DoD's Health and Human Services federal partner, and measures from national professional organizations, can provide benchmarks for both direct and Purchased Care. In particular, NHQM data available on the CMS Hospital Compare website is collected for all participating Purchased Care facilities similar to data collected for direct care. NHQM data is currently used to benchmark Purchased Care and direct care hospital quality performance for the Timely and Effective Care measures against CMS' best performers. Data is reviewed semiannually at a working group and the data files are available to the Managed Care Support Contractors (MCSCs) for additional analysis. Measures used in NHQM comparison contain process, outcome and experience of care measures, as well as several medical conditions. NHQM data is an existing resource that can be leveraged to compare direct and Purchased Care hospital quality performance.

CMS is also in a transitional period for adoption of the CQMC measures. Network providers are not yet required to submit CQMC measures to CMS, although there is much overlap between CQMC measures and measures required through the CMS Quality Payment Program. DHA is coordinating with CMS and the NQF on DoD implementation of CQMC measures. As

CQMC measures are adopted, the DHA can remain proactive and strategic in selection of measures for both direct and Purchased Care comparison.

Recommendation 2: The GAO recommends that the ASD(HA) should establish, as appropriate, performance standards related to the Purchased Care Dashboard measures that are consistent with MHS's performance standards for direct care, ensure they are applied to individual purchased care providers and require corrective actions to be taken when providers do not meet those standards. (Recommendation 2)

DoD Response: The Department concurs with the recommendation.

The DHA agrees with the need to improve accountability of MCSCs to be compliant with established performance standards specific to a set of measures that are collected for both direct and Purchased Care. The DHA plans to improve accountability and promote clinical excellence across both parts of the integrated healthcare delivery system. However, as Purchased Care is a contractual arrangement with the MCSCs, the DHA will hold the contractor to the contractual performance standards, but currently cannot take action against individual providers based solely on performance.

The DHA agrees that measures of individual provider performance should be augmented, and consistent with measures in direct care, where possible. The MCSCs do already collect and use Hospital Compare data. We are committed to a consistent level of high quality care in both the direct and Purchased Care systems. The DHA also concurs with standardizing the use of this data across the system, and collaborating with MCSCs to incentivize high performing facilities and assist those underperforming to improve quality performance. Purchased Care is considering using other sources of quality data such as Leapfrog® data, which is available for a significant majority of private sector hospitals that are utilized by TRICARE beneficiaries.

For individual outpatient provider practices in the Purchased Care network, collecting and utilizing quality performance data that is not reflected in claims in a systematic manner is exceedingly difficult. Although the report recommends using CQMC data, CMS is in the early stages of implementing the program. Once further guidance from CMS is known regarding the reporting structure of CQMC data, TRICARE will work together with the MCSCs to identify prevalence of network providers who report CQMC data to CMS as another method for measuring TRICARE provider performance. Rather than the corrective action approach (except in cases where there is a serious quality event already managed with MCSC-imposed corrective actions), the Department plans to expand its value-based efforts and incentivize providers who meet and exceed quality standards.

In: Defense Health Care
Editor: Frederick Duncan

ISBN: 978-1-53615-175-6

Chapter 2

DEFENSE HEALTH CARE: DOD SHOULD DEMONSTRATE HOW ITS PLAN TO TRANSFER THE ADMINISTRATION OF MILITARY TREATMENT FACILITIES WILL IMPROVE EFFICIENCY*

United States Government Accountability Office

ABBREVIATIONS

DOD	Department of Defense
DHA	Defense Health Agency
MTFs	military treatment facilities
NDAA	National Defense Authorization Act

* This is an edited, reformatted and augmented version of United States Government Accountability Office; Report to Congressional Committees, Publication No. GAO-19-53, dated October 2018.

WHY GAO DID THIS STUDY

In fiscal year 2017, DOD provided health care to 9.4 million beneficiaries, including servicemembers, retirees, and their families at a cost of $43 billion. For more than a decade, partially in response to congressional mandates, DOD has worked to address inefficiencies in the Military Health System to control costs. To further achieve efficiencies, the NDAA for Fiscal Year 2017 required DOD to develop an implementation plan that addressed four elements related to transferring the administration of the MTFs to the DHA. DOD issued the plan in June 2018.

The NDAA also included a provision for GAO to review the plan. GAO determined whether (1) DOD's plan included the statutory elements related to the transfer of administration of the MTFs to the DHA and (2) additional information would be useful to demonstrate that the plan will reduce or better manage duplication and improve efficiencies. GAO assessed DOD's plan against the required elements and, where appropriate, considered the extent to which the plan provided detailed information related to key change management practices identified in past GAO work.

WHAT GAO RECOMMENDS

GAO recommends that DOD define and analyze the 16 operational readiness and installation-specific medical functions for duplication, validate headquarters-level personnel requirements, and identify the least costly mix of personnel. DOD concurred with all three recommendations and noted actions it was taking to address each one.

WHAT GAO FOUND

The Department of Defense's (DOD) June 2018 plan addressed the four statutory elements for the transfer of the administration of the military treatment facilities (MTFs) from the military departments to the Defense Health Agency (DHA). Specifically, the plan provided information on (1) how the DHA will take administrative responsibility of the MTFs; (2) efforts to eliminate duplicative activities; (3) efforts to maximize efficiencies in the DHA's activities; and (4) reductions of headquarters-level military, civilian, and contractor personnel. DOD dedicated most of the plan to describing the governance structure of the proposed administrative framework and to describing the timeline for a phased transfer of the approximately 457 MTFs to the DHA by October 1, 2021. Initially, DOD was to transfer responsibility for the administration of the MTFs to the DHA by October 1, 2018. However, Congress in the National Defense Authorization Act (NDAA) for Fiscal Year 2019 amended the law to allow, among other things, DOD to complete the transfer by September 30, 2021.

DOD has taken key steps in its June 2018 plan to improve the effectiveness and efficiency of the administration of MTFs. However, DOD's plan has two weaknesses that could be mitigated with additional information. Specifically,

- DOD excluded 16 operational readiness and installation-specific medical functions from consideration for transfer to the DHA. DOD did not define or analyze the potential effect of excluding these functions, which include dental care, substance abuse, and occupational health. Senior officials from the DHA and the Assistant Secretary of Defense for Health Affairs acknowledged that transferring the dental care function, for example, from the military departments to the DHA could potentially reduce duplicative activities.
- DOD's plans to achieve the stated goal of reducing headquarters-level personnel, including contractor personnel, by 10 percent are unclear. In its June 2018 plan, DOD states that the DHA will experience personnel growth during each phase of the transition, but that it expects to reduce headquarters-level personnel by 10 percent by 2021. However, the plan does not provide specific details about how DOD will achieve the established goal of reducing

headquarters-level personnel by 10 percent while the DHA experiences personnel growth. Further, the plan does not address whether and how contractor personnel factor into the reduction. This lack of clarity exists because DOD has not validated headquarters-level personnel requirements or conducted a comprehensive review to identify the least costly mix of military, civilian, and contractor personnel to meet the validated requirements.

Until DOD takes action to resolve these two weaknesses, DOD will likely not be well positioned to reduce or better manage duplication and improve efficiencies, including reducing headquarters-level personnel across the Military Health System. Furthermore, Congress will lack important information to determine the extent to which the transfer of the administration of the MTFs to the DHA is being planned and implemented effectively and efficiently.

October 30, 2018

The Honorable James M. Inhofe
Chairman

The Honorable Jack Reed
Ranking Member
Committee on Armed Services
United States Senate

The Honorable Mac Thornberry
Chairman
The Honorable Adam Smith
Ranking Member
Committee on Armed Services
House of Representatives

In fiscal year 2017, the Department of Defense's (DOD) Military Health System provided health care to 9.4 million beneficiaries including servicemembers, retirees, and their family members at a cost of $43 billion.[1] For more than a decade, DOD has worked to address congressional concerns about governance-related inefficiencies in the Military Health System, in part by responding to a number of congressional mandates.[2] For example, in September 2013, DOD established the Defense Health Agency (DHA) to create a more integrated Military Health System and achieve cost savings at headquarters-level organizations by, among other things, streamlining the administrative support for the military departments' respective medical programs.[3] The DHA also assumed the administrative responsibility for managing military treatment facilities (MTFs) in the National Capital Region—specifically, the Walter Reed National Military Medical Center and the Fort Belvoir Community Hospital.[4] According to National Capital Region Medical Directorate information, the DHA exercises authority,

---

[1] Defense Health Agency, *Evaluation of the TRICARE Program: Fiscal Year 2018 Report to Congress, Access, Cost, and Quality Data through Fiscal Year 2017* (Feb. 28, 2018); the cost figure is for the Defense Health Program, including transfers from the Medicare- Eligible Retiree Health Care Fund. Department of Defense, *Defense Health Program Fiscal Year (FY) 2019 Budget Estimates: Operation and Maintenance Procurement Research, Development, Test and Evaluation*, Volume 1: Justification Estimates, Volume. 2: Data Book (Feb. 2018). According to officials with the Office of the Under Secretary of Defense for Personnel and Readiness, the cost figure for the Defense Health Program does not include costs that are funded through other accounts.

[2] The National Defense Authorization Act (NDAA) for Fiscal Year 2013 required that DOD create a detailed plan for carrying out its health care system reform, including goals; performance measures; required personnel levels; and a schedule for carrying out the reform goals, among other things. Pub. L. No. 112-239, § 731 (2013). The NDAA for Fiscal Year 2017 directed the transfer of responsibility for the administration of military medical treatment facilities to the Director of the Defense Health Agency. Pub. L. No. 114-328, § 702 (2016).

[3] Headquarters elements of DHA are considered major DOD headquarters activities. Department of Defense Instruction 5100.73, *Major DOD Headquarters Activities* (Dec. 1, 2007) (incorporating change 2, June 12, 2012).

[4] DHA also has authority, direction, and control over subordinate clinics of the Walter Reed National Military Medical Center and the Fort Belvoir Community Hospital. Department of Defense Directive 5136.13, *Defense Health Agency (DHA)* (Sept. 30, 2013). According to a draft DHA concept of operations, "administration" refers to the responsibility for governing MTFs (i.e., execution of day-to-day operations) and "management" refers to the authority, direction, and control to ensure MTF accountability (i.e., authority, direction and control over the organizational structure and management of functional capabilities within that structure to provide oversight). See *Defense Health Agency Concept of Operations: Transfer of Administration and Management of the Military Medical Treatment Facilities to Defense Health Agency Authority, Direction, and Control*, Version 1.53 (June 7, 2018).

direction, and control over approximately 6 MTFs in the National Capital Region.[5] MTFs, which include military hospitals, ambulatory care clinics, and dental clinics, are part of the direct care system.[6] According to DOD, these MTFs total approximately 679.[7] The direct care system represents health care facilities and medical support organizations owned by DOD and managed by the military departments' respective Surgeons General.[8]

Section 702 of the National Defense Authorization Act (NDAA) for Fiscal Year 2017 amended Chapter 55 of title 10, United States Code, to include a new section entitled "1073c Administration of Defense Health Agency and military medical treatment facilities," which describes how the DHA will take administrative responsibility of the MTFs.[9] According to that section, the Director of the DHA shall be responsible for the administration of each MTF, including with respect to budgetary matters; information technology; and health care administration and management, among other things.[10]

Section 702 of the NDAA for Fiscal Year 2017 required that the Secretary of Defense develop a plan that includes four elements, such as how the Secretary will carry out subsection (a) of section 1073c of title 10 of the United States Code and efforts to eliminate duplicative activities, among others.[11] DOD provided three interim reports to Congress in response to section 702. The first two interim reports, dated March 31, 2017, and June

---

[5] This information also states that the DHA exercises authority, direction, and control over the Joint Pathology Center.

[6] MTFs also include other facilities within the direct care system.

[7] DOD estimated that there are about 679 military hospitals, ambulatory care clinics, and dental clinics in fiscal year 2018. See Defense Health Agency, *Evaluation of the TRICARE Program: Fiscal Year 2018 Report to Congress; Access, Cost, and Quality Data through Fiscal Year 2017* (Feb. 28, 2018).

[8] The Department of the Navy administers health care for the Marine Corps. Air Force Major Commands direct MTF activities; the Air Force Medical Operations Agency supports but does not command Air Force MTFs.

[9] Pub. L. No. 114-328, § 702 (2016).

[10] Section 1073c of title 10, United States Code, was amended by the John S. McCain NDAA for Fiscal Year 2019. Pub. L. No. 115-232, § 711 (2018). Among other things, the amendment requires that the Secretary of Defense establish a timeline to ensure the transfer of MTF administration from the military departments to the DHA no later than September 30, 2021.

[11] Pub. L. No. 114-328, § 702(d) (2016).

30, 2017, were DOD's preliminary draft of the plan.[12] In these reports, DOD discussed its intent to use the "component model" as the administrative framework. Under the component model, the Director of the DHA would administer each MTF through military department-led intermediary component commands and military department-led MTFs. Congress, in the Conference report accompanying the NDAA for Fiscal Year 2018 that was issued in November 2017, raised concern about the component model.[13] The third interim report, which DOD provided to Congress March 30, 2018, did not include the component model as DOD's administrative framework, but provided details on a new proposed framework to transition MTF administration and management to the DHA.[14] According to the third interim report, DOD decided after deeper analysis and discussions with Congress that the component model did not adequately satisfy the requirements of subsection (a) of section 1073c. DOD submitted its final plan (hereinafter referred to as the plan) to Congress on June 28, 2018.[15] Figure 1 provides a timeline of DOD's efforts in response to section 702.

Section 702 also includes a provision for us to review the plan by September 1, 2018.[16] In this chapter, we determined whether (1) DOD's plan included the statutory elements related to the transfer of the administration of the MTFs to the DHA and (2) additional information would be useful to

---

[12] Department of Defense, *Report to the Armed Services Committees of the Senate and House of Representatives, Plan to Implement Section 1073c of Title 10, United States Code, Interim Report – Preliminary Draft* (Mar. 31, 2017) and Department of Defense, *Report to the Armed Services Committees of the Senate and House of Representatives, Plan to Implement Section 1073c of Title 10, United States Code, Second Interim Report* (June 30, 2017). We reported, as required, on DOD's preliminary draft of the plan in September 2017. See *GAO, Defense Health Reform: Steps Taken to Plan the Transfer of the Administration of the Military Treatment Facilities to the Defense Health Agency, but Work Remains to Finalize the Plan*, GAO-17-791R (Washington, D.C.: Sept. 29, 2017).

[13] H.R. Rep. No. 115-404, at 849-850 (2017) (Conf. Rep.).

[14] Department of Defense, *Report to the Armed Services Committees of the Senate and House of Representatives, Preliminary Draft Plan to Implement 1073c of Title 10, United States Code, Interim Report* (Mar. 31, 2018).

[15] Department of Defense, *Report to the Armed Services Committees of the Senate and House of Representatives, Final Plan to Implement Section 1073c of Title 10, United States Code, Final Report* (June. 30, 2018). Section 702 of the NDAA for Fiscal Year 2017 required that DOD provide the final plan to the House and Senate Armed Services Committees no later than March 1, 2018. Pub. L. No. 114-328, § 702(e)(2) (2016).

[16] To meet this requirement, we provided a draft report to the defense congressional committees.

demonstrate that the plan will reduce or better manage duplication and improve efficiencies.

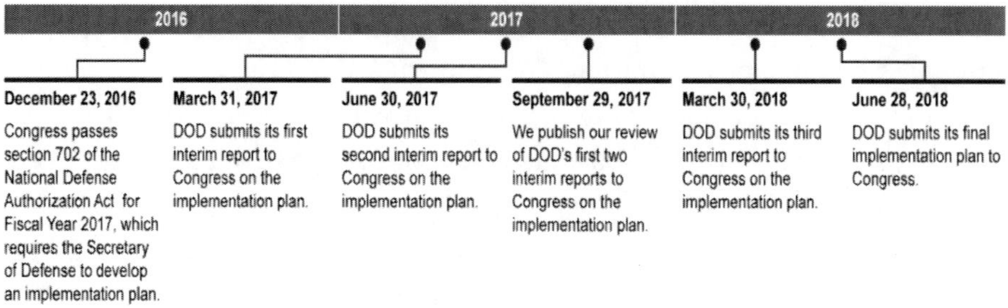

Source: GAO. | GAO-19-53.

Note: Section 702 of the National Defense Authorization Act for Fiscal Year 2017 amended Chapter 55 of title 10, United States Code, to include a new section entitled "1073c Administration of Defense Health Agency and military medical treatment facilities," which describes how the Defense Health Agency will take administrative responsibility of the military treatment facilities. Section 702 also requires that the Secretary of Defense develop a plan that includes four elements, such as how the Secretary will carry out subsection (a) of section 1073c of title 10 of the United States Code and efforts to eliminate duplicative activities.

Figure 1. Timeline of Department of Defense Efforts to Address Section 702 of the National Defense Authorization Act for Fiscal Year 2017.

For objective one, we determined whether DOD's plan included the four elements set forth in the statute.[17] Two analysts independently conducted this assessment and reconciled any differences to reach a consensus on the overall assessment. For objective two, where appropriate, we also considered the extent to which the plan provided detailed information related to key change management practices identified in our prior work, which could help ensure that DOD effectively and efficiently achieves its goals.[18]

---

[17] Pub. L. No. 114-328, § 702(d) (2016).

[18] GAO, *Government Reorganization: Key Questions to Assess Agency Reform Efforts,* GAO-18-427 (Washington, D.C.: June 13, 2018). This chapter identifies key questions that Congress, agencies, and others should consider for the development and implementation of agency reforms, based on our prior work. In the report, the term "reforms" was used to broadly include any organizational changes—such as major transformations, mergers, consolidations, and other reorganizations—and efforts to streamline and improve the efficiency and effectiveness of government operations. Key change management practices described in this chapter are derived from our prior work, such as, but not limited to GAO, *Fragmentation,*

We also reviewed key planning documents identified by DOD in developing the plan and other relevant documents, such as the Under Secretary of Defense for Personnel and Readiness memorandums related to section 702 and concepts of operations from the Assistant Secretary of Defense for Health Affairs; the DHA; and the Army, the Navy, and the Air Force departments.[19]

For both objectives, we corroborated our understanding of the plan by conducting interviews with officials from the Office of the Under Secretary of Defense for Personnel and Readiness; the Office of the Assistant Secretary of Defense for Health Affairs; the DHA; the Health Care Management Reform Team (one of the reform teams created in 2017 by the DOD to address improved mission effectiveness and efficiencies in DOD); the Office of Cost Assessment and Program Evaluation; the Army Medical Command, Office of the Surgeon General and the Office of the Assistant Secretary of the Army Manpower and Reserve Affairs; the Navy Bureau of Medicine and Surgery; the Air Force Medical Service; and the Joint Staff Surgeon.

Overlap, and Duplication: An Evaluation and Management Guide GAO-15-49SP (Washington, D.C.: Apr. 14, 2015) and *Streamlining Government: Key Practices from Select Efficiency Initiatives Should Be Shared Governmentwide*, GAO-11-908 (Washington, D.C.: Sept. 30, 2011). We focused on those change management practices that are particularly relevant to assist DOD in achieving its effort to address statutory requirements in its planning to identify efficiencies, potentially reduce duplicative activities, and achieve personnel reduction goals.

[19] We reviewed the following Under Secretary of Defense for Personnel and Readiness memorandums: *Authorities and Responsibilities of Military Treatment Facility Leaders, Service Leaders and the Military Medical Departments* (Feb. 21, 2018); *Managing the Transformation of the Military Health System* (Mar. 21, 2018); *Construct for Implementation of Section 702* (May 22, 2018); *Manpower Requirements Validation for the Defense Health Agency Headquarters* (June 7, 2018); and *Zero-Based Review of Military Department Medical Manpower* (June 15, 2018). We also reviewed the following documents: the Assistant Secretary of Defense for Health Affairs, *Military Health System Concept of Operations*, Version 9 (2018); the DHA Draft *Defense Health Agency Concept of Operations: Transfer of Administration and Management of Military Medical Treatment Facilities To Defense Health Agency Authority, Direction, and Control,* Version 1.53 (June 7, 2018); the Army Pre-decisional Draft of its *Army Service Concept of Operations, Transfer of Administration and Management of Military Medical Treatment Facilities to Defense Health Agency, Version 26* (May 2018); the Navy Bureau of Medicine and Surgery Draft *Navy Medicine Readiness and Training Commands: Concept of Operations* (May 2018); and the Office of the Air Force Surgeon General Pre-decisional Draft *Air Force Medical Service Operational Readiness Platform Concept of Operations (CONOPS)* (May 23, 2018).

We conducted this performance audit from March 2018 to October 2018 in accordance with generally accepted government auditing standards. Those standards require that we plan and perform the audit to obtain sufficient, appropriate evidence to provide a reasonable basis for our findings and conclusions based on our audit objectives. We believe that the evidence obtained provides a reasonable basis for our findings and conclusions based on our audit objectives.

BACKGROUND

History of Military Health System Reforms

For over a decade, Congress and DOD have led a series of efforts to address the governance structure of the Military Health System, including recommending and implementing significant organizational realignments. DOD undertook a significant organizational realignment effort in June 2011, creating an internal task force to review the governance of the Military Health System and subsequently identified as priorities cost containment, greater integration, and increased unity of effort. In March 2012, DOD submitted a report to Congress that, among other things, proposed creating the DHA to achieve cost savings at headquarters- and administrative-level organizations, TRICARE, the headquarters of military departments' medical commands and agencies, and other management organizations within the Military Health System that do not directly provide health care services.[20] DOD established the DHA in September 2013 to provide administrative support for the military departments' respective medical programs by adopting common clinical and business processes, combining common shared services, and coordinating the work of the military departments'

[20] Through regional contracts, TRICARE administers the purchased care system, which comprises a civilian network of hospitals and providers. Prior to October 1, 2013, the TRICARE Management Activity, an entity within the Department of Defense (DOD), was responsible for overseeing DOD's regionally structured health care program. Upon its establishment, the DHA assumed management responsibility of numerous functions of DOD's medical health system, including the former TRICARE Management Activity.

respective MTFs and care purchased from the private sector.[21] The DHA also assumed the administrative responsibility for managing the MTFs in the National Capital Region.

The NDAA for Fiscal Year 2013 required that DOD create a detailed plan for carrying out its health care system reform to include the goals of the reform and performance measures to achieve them; the personnel levels required for the DHA and the National Capital Region Medical Directorate; and specific information on the shared services, among other things.[22] In 2015, we reported on DOD's establishment of the DHA and made five recommendations, and DOD concurred or partially concurred with all of these recommendations.[23] DOD has implemented two of the five recommendations by completing some baseline personnel assessments of the DHA workforce and reporting the number and cost of administrative headquarters personnel within the Military Health System in DOD's fiscal year 2018 Defense Health Program budget estimates. Of the three open recommendations, two relate directly to assessing personnel requirements within the DHA. As of January 2018, these recommendations have not been fully addressed and remain open because DOD has not established processes and procedures to create an overall personnel management process for the DHA.

In December 2016, Congress expanded the role of the DHA by directing the transfer of responsibility for the administration of each MTF from the military departments to the DHA.[24] Pursuant to section 1073c(a) of title 10, United States Code, the Director of the DHA shall be responsible for the administration of each MTF, including with respect to budgetary matters, information technology, health care administration and management, administrative policy and procedure, military medical construction, and any

[21] According to the DOD, a "shared services concept" is a combination of common services performed across the medical community, such as Medical Logistics; Facility Planning; Medical Education and Training; Health Information Technology; and Medical Research, Development, and Acquisition.

[22] Pub. L. No. 112-239, § 731 (2013).

[23] GAO, *Defense Health Care Reform: Actions Needed to Help Ensure Defense Health Agency Maintains Implementation Progress,* GAO-15-759 (Washington, D.C.: Sept. 10, 2015).

[24] Pub. L. No. 114-328, § 702 (2016).

other matters the Secretary of Defense determines appropriate.[25] Section 702 of the NDAA for Fiscal Year 2017 required that the Secretary of Defense develop a plan to implement section 1073c of title 10, United States Code, that includes the following four elements:[26]

A. how the Secretary will carry out subsection (a) of section 1073c of title 10 of the United States Code;[27]
B. efforts to eliminate duplicative activities carried out by the elements of the DHA and military departments;
C. efforts to maximize efficiencies in the activities carried out by the DHA; and
D. how the Secretary will implement section 1073c in a manner that reduces the number of members of the armed forces, civilian employees who are full-time equivalent employees, and contractors relating to the headquarters activities of the Military Health System, as of the date of the enactment of the act.

Section 702 of the NDAA for Fiscal Year 2017 also included a provision for us to review DOD's interim and final reports on the implementation plan.[28] In our review of DOD's plan in September 2017, we noted that DOD had selected the component model—in which the Director of the DHA would administer each MTF through military department-led intermediary component commands and military department-led MTFs— as the administrative model DOD would use to meet the requirements specified in section 702.[29] Congress, in the Conference report accompanying the NDAA for Fiscal Year 2018 that was issued in November 2017, raised concern about DOD's lack of progress on the development of the plan and about the

---

[25] 10 U.S.C. § 1073c.

[26] The interim report on DOD's preliminary draft of the implementation plan was due by March 1, 2017, and the final report on the implementation plan was due by March 1, 2018.

[27] As previously noted, Chapter 55 of title 10, United States Code, included a new section entitled, "1073c Administration of Defense Health Agency and military medical treatment facilities," which describes how the DHA will take administrative responsibility of the MTFs.

[28] Pub. L. No. 114-328, § 702(e)(3) (2016).

[29] GAO-17-791R.

component model.[30] Specifically, Congress noted that the component model was an attempt to maintain current stove-piped organizational constructs that risk continued inefficiencies in the Military Health System command and governance structure. In the third interim report, DOD found that the component model would not be adequate to satisfy statutory requirements and subsequently changed from the component model to a new administrative framework.[31]

Amendments from the NDAA for Fiscal Year 2019

The NDAA for Fiscal Year 2019 amended section 1073c of title 10, United States Code.[32] The NDAA for Fiscal Year 2019, among other things, provided additional authorities to the Director of the DHA, such as the authority to determine total workforce requirements at each MTF and established within the DHA two subordinate organizations—one for research and development, and one for public health. Additionally, the NDAA for Fiscal Year 2019 extended the date for the transfer of the administration of the MTFs to the DHA from the original deadline of October 1, 2018, to September 30, 2021. Section 1073c of title 10, United States Code, including these amendments, is reproduced in appendix I.

Roles and Responsibilities of Key DOD Entities in the Military Health System

Currently, the Under Secretary of Defense for Personnel and Readiness, the Assistant Secretary of Defense for Health Affairs, the DHA, and the

---

[30] H.R. Rep. No. 115-404 at 849-850 (2017) (Conf. Rep.).

[31] Department of Defense, *Report to the Armed Services Committees of the Senate and House of Representatives, Preliminary Draft Plan to Implement 1073c of Title 10, United States Code, Interim Report* (Mar.31, 2018).

[32] Pub. L. No. 115-232, § 711 (2018).

military departments have various responsibilities for the oversight and management of the Military Health System:

- The Under Secretary of Defense for Personnel and Readiness is the principal staff assistant and advisor to the Secretary and Deputy Secretary of Defense for health affairs and, in that capacity, develops policies, plans, and programs for health and medical affairs.[33]
- The Assistant Secretary of Defense for Health Affairs has the primary responsibility for the Military Health System and serves as the principal advisor to the Under Secretary of Defense for Personnel and Readiness for all DOD health policies, programs, and activities.[34] The Assistant Secretary of Defense for Health Affairs also has the authority to develop policies; conduct analyses; issue guidance; provide advice and make recommendations to the Secretary of Defense, the Under Secretary of Defense for Personnel and Readiness, and others; and provide oversight to the DOD components on matters pertaining to the Military Health System. Further, the Assistant Secretary of Defense for Health Affairs prepares and submits a DOD Unified Medical Program budget[35] to provide resources for the Military Health System.
- The Director of the DHA, in addition to carrying out the responsibilities outlined above, manages the execution of policy developed by the Assistant Secretary of Defense for Health Affairs.[36]

---

[33] Department of Defense Directive 5124.02, *Under Secretary of Defense for Personnel and Readiness (USD(P&R))* (June 23, 2008).

[34] Department of Defense Directive 5136.01, *Assistant Secretary of Defense for Health Affairs (ASD(HA))* (Sept. 30, 2013) (incorporating change 1, effective Aug. 10, 2017).

[35] The DOD Unified Medical Program consists of the Defense Health Program appropriation, the medical military construction appropriation, military personnel funds for military personnel supporting the Military Health System, and the estimated payments to the DOD Medicare-Eligible Retiree Health Care Fund.

[36] DOD Directive 5136.13.

- The Secretaries of the military departments coordinate with the Assistant Secretary of Defense for Health Affairs to develop certain Military Health System policies, standards, and procedures and provide military personnel and other authorized resources to support the activities of the DHA, among other things. The Surgeon General of each military department serves as the principal advisor to the Secretary of the military department concerned on all health and medical matters of the military department.

DOD Addressed the Statutory Elements for the Transfer of the Administration of the MTFs to the DHA

DOD addressed each of the four statutory elements in its June 2018 plan. DOD dedicated most of the plan to describing the governance structure of DOD's new administrative framework and to describing the schedule for the phased transfer of the administration of approximately 457 MTFs to the DHA by October 1, 2021.[37] DOD's plan provided less detail on addressing efforts to eliminate duplicative activities; maximizing efficiency; and reducing the number of headquarters-level military, civilian, and contractor personnel. The following provides a summary of what DOD's plan included for each of the four elements in the statute:

- Information on efforts to transfer the administration of the MTFs to the DHA.[38] In its plan, DOD described the transfer of the MTFs to the DHA, including budgetary matters, information technology, health care administration and management, administrative policy and procedure, military medical construction, and all other MTF

[37] As noted earlier, the NDAA for Fiscal Year 2019 extended the date for the transfer of the administration of the MTFs to the DHA to September 30, 2021.

[38] This section corresponds to how the Secretary will carry out subsection (a) of section 1073c of title 10 of the United States Code. Pub. L No. 114-328, § 702(d)(2)(A) (2016).

operations. DOD dedicated most of the plan to describing the (1) new governance structure of the proposed administrative framework model and (2) timeline for the phased transfer of the administration of the 457 MTFs from the military departments' respective medical commands to the DHA. For example, DOD states that Military Health System governance will shift its focus from consensus-driven bodies that address both policy and management issues to a smaller, streamlined set of oversight councils that focus on high-level, Military Health System-wide policy and budgetary matters. According to the plan, the Assistant Secretary of Defense for Health Affairs will resolve matters that involve both the military departments and the DHA. DOD also stated that the DHA plans to establish six intermediate management organizations (two for each region) to assist with the administration and management of the MTFs, which are broken out as follows: an East Region, a West Region, and outside the United States.[39] Further, DOD stated that the DHA had established an Assistant Director position for Health Care Administration, as well as four Deputy Assistant Director positions for Information Operations, Financial Operations, Health Care Operations, and Medical Affairs.

Regarding the timeline for the phased transfer, beginning no later than October 1, 2018, DOD will transfer 5 of its approximately 679[40] MTFs to the DHA for the first phase of the transition. MTFs transferring to the DHA for the first phase include the Womack Army Medical Center, Fort Bragg; the Naval Hospital Jacksonville; Force 81st Medical Group, Keesler Air Force Base; 4th Medical Group, Seymour Johnson Air Force Base; and 628th Medical

[39] According to the plan, the Director of the DHA will be responsible for the administration of each MTF through DHA-established intermediate management organizations with respect to budgetary matters, information technology, health care administration and management, administrative policy and procedure, military medical construction, and all other MTF operations.

[40] DOD estimated that there are about 679 military hospitals, ambulatory care clinics, and dental clinics in fiscal year 2018. See Defense Health Agency, *Evaluation of the TRICARE Program: Fiscal Year 2018 Report to Congress; Access, Cost, and Quality Data through Fiscal Year 2017* (Feb. 28, 2018).

Group, Joint Base Charleston. In the second phase of the transition, which will begin no later than October 1, 2019, DOD will transfer 244 MTFs from the East Region to the DHA. The third phase will begin no later than October 1, 2020, and will include 134 MTFs from the West Region. The fourth phase will include 79 MTFs outside the United States and begin no later than October 1, 2021. DOD also provided DHA organizational charts for each of the four phases.

- Information on efforts to eliminate duplicative activities carried out by the DHA and the military departments.[41] In its plan, DOD noted that it is undertaking an analysis of the functions that will be performed at DHA headquarters and at the military departments' respective medical department headquarters. In the plan, DOD provided three figures listing the functions, functional responsibilities, and functional requirements that will be carried out by the DHA, the DHA intermediate management organizations, and the military departments' medical department headquarters. Specifically, the functions listed included those functions that should be with the DHA intermediate management organizations, such as Emergency Planning and Preparation, and those functions that should be with the military departments' medical department intermediate commands or headquarters, such as Quality and Safety for Healthcare in the Operational Setting. The three figures primarily focused on functions to be performed during the first phase of the transition.
- Information on efforts to maximize efficiencies in the activities carried out by the DHA.[42] In its plan, DOD included information about its three principle efforts currently underway to address efficiencies. Specifically, DOD describes its broader efforts to

[41] This section corresponds to efforts to eliminate duplicative activities carried out by the elements of the DHA and by the military departments. Pub. L No. 114-328, § 702(d)(2)(B) (2016).

[42] This section corresponds to efforts to maximize efficiencies in the activities carried out by the DHA. Pub. L No. 114-328, § 702(d)(2)(C) (2016).

streamline clinical and business processes across the Military Health System and links some of these broader initiatives to section 702.[43] According to the plan, efforts such as the use of centralized contract support functions and common purchasing, among others, are made possible because of the transfer of the administration of the MTFs to the DHA. Specific to the transfer of MTFs to the DHA as required by section 1073c of title 10 of the United States Code, DOD's plan stated that the DHA is developing, publishing, and implementing procedural instructions to help administer and manage the MTFs. The plan also states that each MTF transferring to the DHA will establish a performance plan—referred to as a quadruple aim performance plan—to monitor performance. According to the plan, Military Health System leadership adopted the quadruple aim performance plan to monitor MTF performance, which they believe will improve performance and contribute to better outcomes and increased efficiencies.[44] The plan states that the performance of all MTFs in the Military Health System will be monitored using the Military Health System quadruple aim performance plan measures beginning October 1, 2018.

- Information on reducing headquarters-level military, civilian, and contractor personnel within the Military Health System.[45] In its plan, DOD noted that it has already programmed a 25-percent reduction in personnel positions aligned to medical headquarters across the

---

[43] These broader reform efforts began in 2017 when the Secretary of Defense first directed DOD's components to conduct a thorough business review. Components were asked to identify viable reform initiatives to make DOD more effective and efficient and achieve the business reforms necessary to restore military lethality and readiness. The Health Care Reform Management Team identified ten initiatives as part of the reform efforts.

[44] The DHA 2017 report to stakeholders states that the Military Health System Quadruple Aim includes increased readiness, better care, better health, and lower cost, which collectively serve as the strategic framework for the Military Health System. See Defense Health Agency, *2017 Stakeholder Report* (2017).

[45] This section corresponds to how the Secretary will implement section 1073c in a manner that reduces the number of members of the armed forces, civilian employees who are full-time equivalent employees, and contractors relating to the headquarters activities of the Military Health System, as of the date of the enactment of the act. Pub. L No. 114-328, § 702(d)(2)(D) (2016).

enterprise.[46] Specific to the transfer of MTFs to the DHA as required by section 1073c of title 10 of the United States Code, DOD states that the DHA will experience personnel growth during each subsequent phase of the transition in order to undertake its new responsibilities. Additionally, the plan states that DOD expects at least a 10-percent reduction (approximately 695 positions from the current baseline) in headquarters military and civilian personnel by the end of the transition. However, the plan does not provide specific details about how it will achieve the 10-percent reduction while the DHA experiences personnel growth during each phase. The plan includes a figure depicting military and civilian full-time equivalent positions for the current baseline of the DHA and the military departments' respective medical department headquarters and intermediate commands. Contractors are also mentioned in the plan at a high level, but without specific data. Additionally, DOD continues to take steps to evaluate personnel requirements. Specifically, according to two June 2018 Under Secretary of Defense for Personnel and Readiness memorandums, DOD is conducting a review and validation of headquarters-level personnel requirements, which we discuss in more depth later in this chapter.[47]

---

[46] According to the Resource Management Decision we reviewed from February 2016, the 25-percent reduction was specific to defense agency and field activity civilian personnel reductions. Specifically, the decision identified reductions to funds and personnel to implement management headquarters civilian reductions. The Resource Management Decision applied to, for example, the Office of the Under Secretary of Defense for Personnel and Readiness; the Army; the Navy; the Air Force; and the Defense Health Agency, among others. Personnel reductions for this effort were to begin in fiscal year 2017.

[47] Under Secretary of Defense for Personnel and Readiness Memorandum, *Manpower Requirements Validation for the Defense Health Agency Headquarters* (June 7, 2018); Under Secretary of Defense for Personnel and Readiness Memorandum, *Zero-Based Review of Military Department Medical Manpower* (June 15, 2018).

Additional Information Would Be Useful to Demonstrate How the Plan Will Reduce or Better Manage Duplication and Improve Efficiencies

DOD's June 2018 plan takes steps toward reducing duplication and improving effectiveness and efficiency, as previously discussed. However, the plan has two weaknesses that could be mitigated with additional information from DOD. Specifically, DOD cannot be reasonably assured that its plan will reduce or better manage duplication and improve efficiency since (1) certain functions are excluded from the transfer to the DHA and (2) it is unclear, based on the information in the plan and supporting planning documents, how implementation of the plan will result in the achievement of the stated goal of reducing headquarters-level personnel, including contractor personnel, by 10 percent.

DOD Excluded Certain Functions from the Planned Transfer to the DHA That Could Reduce or Better Manage Duplication

As part of its approach for addressing the requirements of section 702 of the NDAA for Fiscal Year 2017, DOD excluded 16 medical functions from the transfer to the DHA. In a February 2018 Under Secretary of Defense for Personnel and Readiness memorandum, these functions were identified as being related to operational readiness and installation- specific missions.[48] That memorandum and another memorandum from the Under Secretary of Defense for Personnel Readiness dated May 2018 listed 16 functions that DOD identified as operational readiness and installation-

[48] Under Secretary of Defense for Personnel and Readiness Memorandum, *Authorities and Responsibilities of Military Treatment Facility Leaders, Service Leaders and the Military Medical Departments* (Feb. 21, 2018).

specific medical functions and that would therefore be excluded from the planned transfer to the DHA (see Table 1).[49]

Table 1. Functions DOD Excluded from the Planned Transfer to the Defense Health Agency

16 Functions to be Excluded	
1. Occupational health	9. Animal medicine
2. Environmental health	10. Dental care (except for oral and maxillofacial surgery)
3. Substance abuse programs	11. Installation emergency response
4. Food protection	12. Deployment-related functions
5. Aerospace physiology	13. Drug demand reduction
6. Aerospace medicine (specifically, non-military treatment facility health care for aviation personnel)	14. Medical logistics for operational units
7. Bioenvironmental engineering	15. Embedded behavioral health
8. Nuclear power and other personnel reliability programs	16. Military aeromedical evacuation (patient movement)

Source: GAO analysis of Department of Defense information. | GAO-19-53.

Note: These functions were identified as operational readiness and installation-specific medical functions and were listed in the following two Under Secretary of Defense for Personnel and Readiness memorandums: *Authorities and Responsibilities of Military Treatment Facility Leaders, Service Leaders and the Military Medical Departments* (Feb. 21, 2018) and *Construct for Implementation of Section 702* (May 22, 2018).

DOD cannot be reasonably assured that its plans are reducing or better managing duplication because DOD has not defined the functions or analyzed the potential for the 16 functions to be transferred to the DHA.[50]

---

[49] Under Secretary of Defense for Personnel and Readiness Memorandum, *Authorities and Responsibilities of Military Treatment Facility Leaders, Service Leaders and the Military Medical Departments* (Feb. 21, 2018); Under Secretary of Defense for Personnel and Readiness Memorandum, *Construct for Implementation of Section 702* (May 22, 2018). These memorandums did not identify all the medical functions being transferred to the DHA.

[50] June 2018 meeting minutes concerning DOD's transition efforts highlighted that DOD was considering analyzing the 16 functions. This analysis would be a part of DOD's review and validation of headquarters-level personnel requirements in response to the June 2018 Under Secretary of Defense for Personnel and Readiness memorandums. Under Secretary of Defense for Personnel and Readiness Memorandum, *Manpower Requirements Validation for*

These functions are not defined in the February or May 2018 memorandums or DOD's plan. The two memorandums list only the functions and state that they are separate from MTF health care delivery services and MTF business operations. One of the memorandums explains that these functions are tied to organizing, training, and equipping personnel for operational readiness missions.[51] These memorandums also do not explain the rationale used to determine that the 16 functions were different from the other MTF health care functions DOD plans to transfer to the DHA. Further, DOD did not provide any analysis or documentation regarding the decision to exclude these 16 functions in the supporting documentation that we reviewed, such as in the concepts of operations for the Assistant Secretary of Defense for Health Affairs, the DHA, the Army, the Navy, and the Air Force. According to senior-level officials from the Assistant Secretary of Defense for Health Affairs and the DHA, there was no formal analysis or documentation to support the decision.

With respect to the exclusion of the transfer of the dental care function to the DHA, Assistant Secretary of Defense for Health Affairs and DHA senior-level officials stated that dental clinics serve only servicemembers, not retirees or family member beneficiaries. Therefore, dental care was considered to be an operational readiness function rather than a health care delivery function, according to these same officials.[52] However, this statement is not completely in line with DOD information regarding overseas dental care and family member beneficiaries. According to DOD information regarding dental care overseas, family members of active- duty

the Defense Health Agency Headquarters (June 7, 2018); Under Secretary of Defense for Personnel and Readiness Memorandum, *Zero-Based Review of Military Department Medical Manpower* (June 15, 2018). According to the memorandums, the reports from the review and validation are required to be completed no later than September 1, 2018. The Office of the Under Secretary of Defense for Personnel and Readiness issued the report on DHA personnel requirements in September 2018. See Office of the Under Secretary of Defense for Personnel and Readiness, *Defense Health Agency: Manpower Requirements Assessment Report* (Sept. 2018).

51 Under Secretary of Defense for Personnel and Readiness Memorandum, *Authorities and Responsibilities of Military Treatment Facility Leaders, Service Leaders and the Military Medical Departments* (Feb. 21, 2018).

52 The Military Health System is responsible for the overall oral health and readiness of servicemembers—both in the active-duty and reserve components. Active-duty servicemembers get most dental care from military dental clinics.

servicemembers can receive dental care from military dental clinics. As such, in some instances the delivery of dental care is not solely for ensuring the readiness of servicemembers. Further, senior-level officials from the Assistant Secretary of Defense for Health Affairs and the DHA acknowledged that transferring the dental care function from the military departments to the DHA could potentially reduce duplicative activities and result in more efficiencies. According to a senior-level DHA official, splitting health care and dental care results in two separate health care delivery organizations.

Across the Military Health System there are approximately 247 (200 in the United States) dental clinics, which represent about a third of DOD's facilities within the direct care system when including dental clinics, military hospitals, and ambulatory care clinics (i.e., approximately 679 facilities in total).[53] Moreover, senior-level officials from the Assistant Secretary of Defense for Health Affairs and the DHA stated that by transferring a function from the military departments to the DHA, DOD reduces the number of managers of a function from four (i.e., at the Army, the Navy, the Air Force, and the DHA) to only one at the DHA.

In our prior work, we have reported that agencies can act to improve the efficiency of their programs by maximizing the level of services provided for a given level of resources, as well as improving programs' effectiveness in achieving their objectives.[54] In particular, we have highlighted the need for agencies to define their mission, functions, activities, services, and processes when identifying fragmentation, overlap, and duplication among programs. Agencies should also assess how, if at all, the fragmented, overlapping, or duplicative functions are related and how they are being coordinated between agencies. Understanding this relationship will help inform decisions about whether and how to increase efficiency or reduce or better manage fragmentation, overlap, or duplication. Also, agencies should assess whether potential effects in areas such as program implementation,

---

[53] Included in DOD's estimate for the 679 facilities are military hospitals, ambulatory care clinics, and dental clinics in fiscal year 2018. See Defense Health Agency, *Evaluation of the TRICARE Program: Fiscal Year 2018 Report to Congress; Access, Cost, and Quality Data through Fiscal Year 2017* (Feb. 28, 2018).

[54] GAO-18-427 and GAO-15-49SP.

outcomes, and costs are positive or negative. Identifying the positive and negative effects of fragmentation, overlap, or duplication will help agencies determine whether or not actions to reduce or better manage the fragmentation, overlap, or duplication are economical and efficient.

However, DOD has not fully determined whether opportunities exist to achieve additional savings due to the lack of analysis, including clear definitions, of the 16 functions that were excluded by DOD. According to senior-level officials from the Assistant Secretary of Defense for Health Affairs and the DHA, there are potential savings by transferring the 16 functions to the DHA, but these have not been adequately analyzed. Without defining and analyzing the 16 functions, DOD cannot assure decisionmakers that it has fully considered all opportunities for reducing or better managing duplication in its plan to transfer the administration of the MTFs to the DHA.

DOD Has Not Demonstrated That Its Plan Will Lead to Reductions in Headquarters Personnel

As previously discussed, DOD's plan identifies the functions that will transfer to the DHA. However, DOD's plan and supporting documents do not provide details on how DOD established the 10-percent reduction of headquarters-level military, civilian, and contractor personnel by 2021, when the administration of the 457 MTFs is to have been transferred to DHA. The plan also states that DHA personnel will grow during each subsequent phase of the transition. Further, information in other related supporting documentation indicates that headquarters-level personnel will increase rather than decrease to achieve the 10-percent reduction goal. Lastly, DOD did not include information in the plan or in its supporting documents concerning contractor personnel reductions.

Officials from the Army, the Navy, the Air Force, the DHA, and the Office of Cost Assessment and Program Evaluation could not identify for us what office within DOD established the 10-percent reduction goal. Our review of key planning documents—the concepts of operations for the Assistant Secretary of Defense for Health Affairs, the DHA, the Army, the

Navy, and the Air Force—found that these documents also did not provide details for the 10-percent reduction of headquarters personnel. Specifically, although these documents included some information regarding personnel reductions, they did not include specific details concerning the 10-percent reduction of headquarters personnel.

DOD states in the plan that the DHA will experience incremental growth in staffing during each phase of the transition in order to undertake its new responsibilities, but does not explain how it will achieve its 10-percent reduction goal given the projected growth. Further, DOD does not provide any data in the plan about how much the DHA will grow during each phase. Senior-level officials from the offices of the Assistant Secretary of Defense for Health Affairs and the DHA stated that there were no explicit restrictions in section 702 of the NDAA for Fiscal Year 2017 that would prohibit the DHA from increasing its number of personnel. However, section 702 does require that the Secretary implement section 1073c in a manner that reduces the number of members of the armed forces; civilian employees who are full-time equivalent employees; and contractors relating to the headquarters activities of the military health system, which includes the DHA.

Further, the projected growth described in DOD's plan is also consistent with a June 2018 DHA pre-decisional draft briefing concerning full-time equivalent positions based on current information provided by the military departments, which describes a transfer of personnel to the DHA from the military departments rather than a reduction in personnel. According to the briefing, full-time equivalents to support future DHA headquarters and intermediate management organizations would not lead to any reductions in personnel. On the contrary, the briefing states that full-time equivalents for military and civilian personnel would increase by 38 percent at the DHA and result in additional costs. A senior-level DHA official confirmed that the information in the briefing relates to a transfer of personnel from the military headquarters to the DHA for health care delivery, not a reduction in personnel that would result in no cost savings. The briefing also states that information related to current and future state full-time equivalent positions is misleading because contractor data, as well as other relevant personnel data, are not included.

Regarding contractor data, DOD did not include any detailed information related to the reduction of contractor personnel in the plan. Specifically, information concerning contractor personnel reductions was not included in the figure or other parts of the section concerning headquarters-level personnel reductions. Overall, contractors are referenced only five times in the entire plan:

- Three of the references are simply repeating the language from the statutory requirement.
- Another reference reiterates that the DHA will assume management responsibilities for civilian and contractor personnel performing health care delivery functions and operations.
- The last reference from the section of the plan related to personnel reductions states that DOD is planning for headquarters personnel reductions, to include military, civilian, and contractor personnel.

In reviewing the concepts of operations for the Assistant Secretary of Defense for Health Affairs, the DHA, the Army, the Navy, and the Air Force for details on contractor personnel, we found that most of these documents did not provide details regarding contractors. Four out of five of the aforementioned concepts of operations did not include information concerning contractors in the context of personnel reductions. Although the Assistant Secretary of Defense for Health Affairs' concept of operations does include information about contractors in the context of personnel reductions, the information does not provide further details about DOD's plans for this effort.

According to DOD Directive 1100.4, *Guidance for Manpower Management*, it is DOD policy that personnel requirements are driven by workload and shall be established at the minimum levels necessary to accomplish mission and performance objectives.[55] This directive states that personnel is a resource and that changes in personnel shall be preceded by changes to the programs, missions, and functions that require personnel

[55] Department of Defense Directive 1100.4, *Guidance for Manpower Management* (Feb. 12, 2005).

resources. Additionally, the directive states that assigned missions shall be accomplished using the least costly mix of personnel (military, civilian, and contract) consistent with military requirements, among other considerations. The directive also states that military (active and reserve) and civilian manpower resources shall be programmed in accordance with validated personnel requirements, among others. Moreover, key change management practices concerning workforce reductions state that before implementing workforce reduction strategies, it is critical that agencies carefully consider how to strategically downsize the workforce and maintain the staff resources to carry out its mission.[56] These same key change management practices also define "efficiency" as maintaining federal government services or outcomes using fewer resources (such as time and money) or improving or increasing the quality or quantity of services or outcomes while maintaining (or reducing) resources.[57]

However, DOD's ability to develop an analytically-based goal for personnel reductions associated with the transfer of administration to DHA, a plan to achieve that goal given that it is projecting growth in personnel, and how contractors factor into its plan has been limited for two reasons. First, DOD has not validated headquarters-level personnel requirements. Second, DOD has not conducted a comprehensive review—a review that, per DOD's own guidance, would involve establishing at minimum levels the requirements necessary to accomplish mission and performance objectives and reflect the consideration of the least costly mix of personnel (i.e., military, civilian and contract) consistent with military requirements, among other considerations, to meet the validated requirements.[58]

Senior-level officials from the offices of the Assistant Secretary of Defense for Health Affairs and the DHA stated that information regarding contractor personnel reductions was not included in the plan because DOD probably did not have these data. These same officials said that it is difficult to obtain contractor personnel data.[59] As we previously noted, DOD has

[56] GAO-18-427.
[57] GAO-18-427 and GAO-11-908.
[58] DOD Directive 1100.4.
[59] Senate Report 114-49, accompanying a bill for the NDAA for Fiscal Year 2016, included a provision for DOD to report on the results of a study comparing the costs of functions

faced challenges with understanding DHA headquarters personnel requirements and composition. In 2015, we reported on DOD's establishment of the DHA and on how, among other things, DOD could not determine DHA's effect on Military Health System administrative and headquarters personnel levels. We found that the DHA had not completed the personnel requirements assessment process or developed a baseline estimate of personnel in the Military Health System before the DHA was created. As discussed previously, we made five recommendations, with which DOD concurred or partially concurred. As of January 2018, DOD had not taken action to fully address three of these recommendations. Of the three recommendations that had not been fully addressed, two relate directly to DHA personnel requirements. Specifically, we recommended the following:

- To provide decision makers with appropriate and more complete information on the continuing implementation, management, and oversight of the DHA, the Secretary of Defense should direct the Assistant Secretary of Defense for Health Affairs to develop a comprehensive requirements assessment process that accounts for needed future skills through the consideration of potential organizational changes and helps ensure appropriate consideration of workforce composition through the determination of the final status of military personnel within the DHA.

---

performed by federal civilians and service contractor personnel at selected installations, among other things. The provision included specific elements for DOD to report, such as an accounting of the full cost of federal civilian and service contractor personnel at the selected installations. S. Rep. No. 114-49, at 223-224 (2015). In April 2018, we reported that DOD's April 2017 report addressed most of the reporting elements, but had only partially addressed the reporting element related to the accounting of the full cost of federal civilian and service contractor personnel. Specifically, we found that DOD had excluded certain non-labor costs from its cost calculations. According to DOD's report, identifying service contractor full-time equivalents is a significant challenge because the level of detail available in each contract varied such that DOD could not employ a single methodology and, unlike federal civilian pay data, there is no centralized database on service-contractor pay. DOD reported that contracts are rarely written to address the cost- per-contractor as a full-time equivalent, and some contracts do not differentiate between labor and non-labor costs. See GAO, *Civilian and Contractor Workforces: DOD's Cost Comparisons Addressed Most Report Elements but Excluded Some Costs*, GAO-18-399 (Washington, D.C.: Apr.17, 2018).

- To provide decision makers with appropriate and more complete information on the continuing implementation, management, and oversight of the DHA, the Secretary of Defense should direct the Assistant Secretary of Defense (Health Affairs) to develop a plan for reassessing and revalidating personnel requirements as the missions and needs of the DHA evolve over time.

Since the recommendations concerning DHA personnel requirements have not been fully addressed and DHA is in the middle of a significant organizational change, it would be timely for DOD to validate headquarters-level personnel requirements and conduct a comprehensive review to determine the appropriate mix of personnel. This validation and comprehensive review should occur prior to transferring authority, direction, and control of the MTFs to the DHA for the third phase, which, as previously noted, is scheduled to begin no later than October 1, 2020.

In June 2018, DOD directed a review and validation of headquarters-level personnel requirements. The Under Secretary of Defense for Personnel and Readiness issued two memorandums concerning the review of headquarters-level personnel requirements.[60] The June 7, 2018, memorandum directs the establishment of cross-service manpower teams to conduct a baseline review of DHA headquarters' current and future personnel requirements. Similarly, the June 15, 2018, memorandum directs the establishment of a working group to determine the appropriate manning of all above MTF-level medical activities in the military departments. This memorandum also requires the working group to review and validate the results of the cross-services manpower teams' assessment of DHA headquarters activities, among other requirements.

---

[60] Under Secretary of Defense for Personnel and Readiness Memorandum, *Manpower Requirements Validation for the Defense Health Agency Headquarters* (June 7, 2018); Under Secretary of Defense for Personnel and Readiness Memorandum, *Zero-Based Review of Military Department Medical Manpower* (June 15, 2018). According to the memorandums, the reports from the review and validation are required to be completed no later than September 1, 2018. The Office of the Under Secretary of Defense for Personnel and Readiness issued the report on DHA personnel requirements in September 2018. See Office of the Under Secretary of Defense for Personnel and Readiness, *Defense Health Agency: Manpower Requirements Assessment Report* (Sept. 2018).

Officials with the Office of the Under Secretary of Defense for Personnel and Readiness involved in these efforts said that the goal of the current review is to identify the DHA's current and future baseline personnel requirements. However, according to these same officials, the review will not (1) validate personnel requirements because of time constraints, (2) identify potential personnel reductions, or (3) consider workforce composition. These officials also clarified that a comprehensive personnel requirements study would take a considerable amount of time and would generate more technical estimates of the work being performed. They said such a study would review major functions and subfunctions, as well as get down to the task level and analyze work processes, which would allow for making process improvement suggestions.

In September 2018, the Office of the Under Secretary of Defense for Personnel and Readiness issued the report on DHA's personnel requirements.[61] The report stated that DHA personnel requirements would increase to support an expanded mission and included several recommendations one of which was to conduct a military essentiality review of DHA positions and functions. According to officials with the Office of the Under Secretary of Defense for Personnel and Readiness, each military department provided headquarters personnel data, which will be reviewed as part of the upcoming Program Budget Review cycle.

Until DOD validates headquarters-level personnel requirements and conducts a comprehensive review that considers the least costly mix of personnel, DOD may not be able to achieve its goal of reducing headquarters-level personnel by 10 percent while maintaining the efficient and effective provision of healthcare services. Furthermore, Congress will lack important information to determine the extent to which the transfer of the administration of the MTFs to the DHA is being planned and implemented effectively and efficiently.

---

[61] According to the report, manpower teams that included representatives from the Army, Navy, and Air Force assessed DHA's baseline and projected future workloads (which considered a future state excluding the 16 operational readiness and installation-specific medical functions and a future state including the 16 functions), among other things. Office of the Under Secretary of Defense for Personnel and Readiness, *Defense Health Agency: Manpower Requirements Assessment Report* (Sept. 2018).

CONCLUSION

Congress required DOD to provide a plan to transfer the administration of the MTFs from the military departments to the DHA. DOD provided a final implementation plan, which made significant changes to the administrative approach described in two of DOD's initial interim plans. In its final plan, DOD addressed all of the elements of the statute. However, the plan did not provide details to demonstrate how DOD will reduce duplicative activities or headquarters-level personnel. Without defining and analyzing the 16 functions currently excluded from transfer to the DHA, validating headquarters-level personnel requirements, and conducting a comprehensive review to determine, per DOD guidance, the least costly mix of personnel, DOD and congressional decisionmakers are not positioned to know how, whether, and to what extent undertaking this significant reform effort will improve effectiveness and efficiency in the administration of the MTFs.

RECOMMENDATIONS FOR EXECUTIVE ACTION

We are making the following three recommendations to the DOD:

1. The Secretary of Defense should ensure that the Assistant Secretary of Defense for Health Affairs, in coordination with Director of the DHA and the Surgeons General of the military departments, define and analyze the 16 operational readiness and installation-specific medical functions currently excluded from transfer to the DHA to determine whether opportunities exist to reduce or better manage duplicative functions and improve efficiencies in the administration of the MTFs. (Recommendation 1)
2. The Secretary of Defense should ensure that the Assistant Secretary of Defense for Health Affairs, in coordination with DHA Assistant Director for Health Care Administration and the Secretaries of the

military departments, validate headquarters-level personnel requirements to determine that they are established at the minimum levels necessary— per DOD guidance—to accomplish missions and achieve objectives before transferring authority, direction, and control of the MTFs to the DHA for the third phase. (Recommendation 2)

3. The Secretary of Defense should ensure that the Assistant Secretary of Defense for Health Affairs, in coordination with DHA Assistant Director for Health Care Administration and the Secretaries of the military departments, conduct a comprehensive review to identify the least costly mix—per DOD guidance—of military, civilian, and contractors needed to meet validated requirements—that is, to perform the functions identified at the DHA headquarters and intermediate management organizations and at the military departments' headquarters and intermediate commands. Additionally, this comprehensive review should be completed before transferring authority, direction, and control of the MTFs to the DHA for the third phase. (Recommendation 3)

AGENCY COMMENTS AND OUR EVALUATION

In written comments reproduced in appendix II, DOD concurred with all three recommendations and noted the actions it was taking to address each recommendation.

In response to our third recommendation, DOD noted that it has completed an extensive review of manpower requirements for the management structure of the DHA. The September 2018 report by the Office of the Under Secretary of Defense for Personnel and Readiness is a first step toward addressing our recommendation. The report provided initial information concerning DHA's personnel requirements. As we noted in our report, however, DOD needs to identify the least costly mix—per DOD guidance—of military, civilian, and contractors once it has validated requirements for DHA.

As an additional comment, DOD noted that since our draft report was provided for comment it has refined the estimated projected growth in full-time equivalents for military and civilian personnel at the DHA from 38 percent to 14 percent. In its comments, DOD stated that it continues to believe that it will achieve a 10 percent reduction. However, as we stated in this chapter, DOD has not demonstrated the extent to which its plan to transfer the MTFs to the DHA will lead to reductions in headquarters-level personnel.

We are sending copies of this chapter to the appropriate congressional committees. We are also sending copies to the Secretary of Defense; the Under Secretary of Defense for Personnel and Readiness; the Assistant Secretary of Defense for Health Affairs; the Director, Cost Assessment and Program Evaluation; the Director, Defense Health Agency; the Surgeon General of the Army; the Surgeon General of the Navy; and the Surgeon General of the Air Force.

Brenda S. Farrell
Director, Defense Capabilities and Management

APPENDIX I: SECTION 1073C OF TITLE 10, UNITED STATES CODE

The National Defense Authorization Act (NDAA) for Fiscal Year 2017 amended Chapter 55 of title 10, United States Code to include a new section: § 1073c Administration of Defense Health Agency and military medical treatment facilities. Section 1073c of title 10, United States Code, as amended by Pub. L. No. 115-91, §§ 713, 1081 (2017), and Pub. L. No. 115-232, § 711 (2018) reads as follows:

§ 1073c. Administration of Defense Health Agency and Military Medical Treatment Facilities

a) Administration of military medical treatment facilities.
   1) In accordance with paragraph (4), by not later than September 30, 2021, the Director of the Defense Health Agency shall be responsible for the administration of each military medical treatment facility, including with respect to--
      A. budgetary matters;
      B. information technology;
      C. health care administration and management;
      D. administrative policy and procedure;
      E. military medical construction; and
      F. any other matters the Secretary of Defense determines appropriate.
   2) In addition to the responsibilities set forth in paragraph (1), the Director of the Defense Health Agency shall, commencing when the Director begins to exercise responsibilities under that paragraph, have the authority—
      A. to direct, control, and serve as the primary rater of the performance of commanders or directors of military medical treatment facilities;
      B. to direct and control any intermediary organizations between the Defense Health Agency and military medical treatment facilities;
      C. to determine the scope of medical care provided at each military medical treatment facility to meet the military personnel readiness requirements of the senior military operational commander of the military installation;
      D. to determine total workforce requirements at each military medical treatment facility;

E. to direct joint manning at military medical treatment facilities and intermediary organizations;
F. to address personnel staffing shortages at military medical treatment facilities; and
G. to select among service nominations for commanders or directors of military medical treatment facilities.

3) The military commander or director of each military medical treatment facility shall be responsible for-
A. ensuring the readiness of the members of the armed forces and civilian employees at such facility; and
B. furnishing the health care and medical treatment provided at such facility.

4) The Secretary of Defense shall establish a timeline to ensure that each Secretary of a military department transitions the administration of military medical treatment facilities from such Secretary to the Director of the Defense Health Agency pursuant to paragraph (1) by the date specified in such paragraph.

5) The Secretary of Defense shall establish within the Defense Health Agency a professional staff to provide policy, oversight, and direction to carry out paragraphs (1) and (2). The Secretary shall carry out this paragraph by appointing the positions specified in subsections (b) and (c).

b) DHA Assistant Director.

1) There is in the Defense Health Agency an Assistant Director for Health Care Administration. The Assistant Director shall--
A. be a career appointee within the Department; and
B. report directly to the Director of the Defense Health Agency.

2) The Assistant Director shall be appointed from among individuals who have equivalent education and experience as a chief executive officer leading a large, civilian health care system.

3) The Assistant Director shall be responsible for the following:
   A. Establishing priorities for health care administration and management.
   B. Establishing policies, procedures, and direction for the provision of direct care at military medical treatment facilities.
   C. Establishing priorities for budgeting matters with respect to the provision of direct care at military medical treatment facilities.
   D. Establishing policies, procedures, and direction for clinic management and operations at military medical treatment facilities.
   E. Establishing priorities for information technology at and between the military medical treatment facilities.

c) DHA Deputy Assistant Directors.
   1) A. There is in the Defense Health Agency a Deputy Assistant Director for Information Operations.
      B. The Deputy Assistant Director for Information Operations shall be responsible for policies, management, and execution of information technology operations at and between the military medical treatment facilities.
   2) A. There is in the Defense Health Agency a Deputy Assistant Director for Financial Operations.
      B. The Deputy Assistant Director for Financial Operations shall be responsible for the policy, procedures, and direction of budgeting matters and financial management with respect to the provision of direct care across the military health system.
   3) A. There is in the Defense Health Agency a Deputy Assistant Director for Health Care Operations.
      B. The Deputy Assistant Director for Health Care Operations shall be responsible for the policy, procedures, and direction

of health care administration in the military medical treatment facilities.

4) A. There is in the Defense Health Agency a Deputy Assistant Director for Medical Affairs.

   B. The Deputy Assistant Director for Medical Affairs shall be responsible for policy, procedures, and direction of clinical quality and process improvement, patient safety, infection control, graduate medical education, clinical integration, utilization review, risk management, patient experience, and civilian physician recruiting.

5) Each Deputy Assistant Director appointed under paragraphs (1) through (4) shall report directly to the Assistant Director for Health Care Administration.

d) Certain responsibilities of DHA Director.

1) In addition to the other duties of the Director of the Defense Health Agency, the Director shall coordinate with the Joint Staff Surgeon to ensure that the Director most effectively carries out the responsibilities of the Defense Health Agency as a combat support agency under section 193 of this title.

2) The responsibilities of the Director shall include the following:

   A. Ensuring that the Defense Health Agency meets the operational needs of the commanders of the combatant commands.

   B. Coordinating with the military departments to ensure that the staffing at the military medical treatment facilities supports readiness requirements for members of the armed forces and health care personnel.

   C. Ensuring that the Defense Health Agency meets the military medical readiness requirements of the senior military operational commanders of the military installations.

e) Additional DHA Organizations.—Not later than September 30, 2022, the Secretary of Defense shall, acting though the Director of the Defense Health Agency, establish within the Defense Health Agency the following:
   1) A subordinate organization, to be called the Defense Health Agency Research and Development—
      A. led, at the election of the Director, by a director or commander (to be called the Director or Commander of Defense Health Agency Research and Development);
      B. comprised of the Army Medical Research and Materiel Command and such other medical research organizations and activities of the armed forces as the Secretary considers appropriate; and
      C. responsible for coordinating funding for Defense Health Program Research, Development, Test, and Evaluation, the Congressionally Directed Medical Research Program, and related Department of Defense medical research.
   2) A subordinate organization, to be called the Defense Health Agency Public Health—
      A. led, at the election of the Director, by a director or commander (to be called the Director or Commander of Defense Health Agency Public Health); and
      B. comprised of the Army Public Health Command, the Navy–Marine Corps Public Health Command, Air Force public health programs, and any other related defense health activities that the Secretary considers appropriate, including overseas laboratories focused on preventive medicine, environmental health, and similar matters.

f) Definitions. In this section:
   1) The term "career appointee" has the meaning given that term in section 3132(a)(4) of title 5.
   2) The term "Defense Health Agency" means the Defense Agency established pursuant to Department of Defense Directive 5136.13, or such successor Defense Agency.

APPENDIX II: COMMENTS FROM THE DEPARTMENT OF DEFENSE

OFFICE OF THE ASSISTANT SECRETARY OF DEFENSE

1200 DEFENSE PENTAGON
WASHINGTON, DC 20301-1200

HEALTH AFFAIRS

SEP 2 5 2018

Ms. Brenda S. Farrell
Director, Defense Capabilities and Management
U.S. Government Accountability Office
441 G Street, NW
Washington DC 20548

Dear Ms. Farrell:

This is the Department of Defense (DoD) response to the Government Accountability Office (GAO) Draft Report, GAO-19-53SU, "DEFENSE HEALTH CARE: DOD Should Demonstrate How Its Plan to Transfer the Administration of Military Treatment Facilities Will Improve Efficiency," dated August 31, 2018 (GAO Code 102682).

Sincerely,

Tom McCaffery
Principal Deputy Assistant Secretary of Defense
for Health Affairs

GOVERNMENT ACCOUNTABILITY OFFICE (GAO) DRAFT REPORT
DATED AUGUST 31, 2018
GAO-19-53SU (GAO CODE 102682)

"DEFENSE HEALTH CARE: DOD Should Demonstrate How Its Plan to Transfer the Administration of Military Treatment Facilities Will Improve Efficiency"

DEPARTMENT OF DEFENSE COMMENTS
TO THE GAO RECOMMENDATIONS

RECOMMENDATION #1:

The Secretary of Defense should ensure that the Assistant Secretary of Defense for Health Affairs, in coordination with Director of the Defense Health Agency (DHA) and the Surgeon General of the military departments, define and analyze the 16 operational readiness and installation-specific medical functions currently excluded from transfer to the DHA to determine whether opportunities exist to reduce or better manage duplicative functions and improve efficiencies in the administration of the MTFs.

Department of Defense (DoD) RESPONSE: Concur. The Department is actively assessing the 16 operational readiness and installation-specific medical functions previously identified for exclusion from transfer to the DHA with the intent of determining the allocation of functions and activities between the Services and the DHA, consistent with revised statutory requirements. This assessment includes representatives from the Services and DHA and will be reviewed through the established transition process.

RECOMMENDATION #2:

The Secretary of Defense should ensure that the Assistant Secretary of Defense for Health Affairs, in coordination with DHA Assistant Director for Health Care Administration and the Secretaries of the military departments validate headquarters-level personnel requirements to determine that they are established at the minimum levels necessary-per DoD guidance-to accomplish missions and achieve objective before transferring authority, direction, and control of MTFs to the DHA for the third phase.

DoD RESPONSE: Concur. The Department is reviewing missions/functions which will transfer from the Services to the DHA and ensuring these functional transitions are fully-synchronized with the Services and DHA. Manpower requirements are being addressed as well, to ensure DHA has the resources needed to meet the requirements of law and DoD policy.

RECOMMENDATION #3:

The Secretary of Defense should ensure that the Assistant Secretary of Defense for Health Affairs, in coordination with the DHA Assistant Director for Health Care Administration and the Secretaries of the military department conduct a comprehensive review to identify the least costly mix-per DOD guidance-of military, civilian, and contractors needed to meet validated requirements-that is, to perform the functions identified at the DHA headquarters and intermediate management organizations and at the military departments' headquarters and intermediate commands. Additionally, this comprehensive review should be completed before transferring authority, direction, and control of the MTFs to the DHA for the third phase.

DoD RESPONSE: Concur. The Department has completed an extensive review of the manpower requirements for the management structure of the DHA. This review was led and conducted by a team composed of manpower professionals outside the DHA, in order to render an objective requirement. The Department is using this data in conjunction with Service inputs to inform programming actions for Fiscal Year 2020. Manpower mix will be evaluated throughout the transition process, optimizing the mix to maximize effectiveness and efficiency.

ADDITIONAL COMMENTS:

The Department would like to provide additional clarification for GAO's statement, "DoD is projecting a growth of 38 percent" on page 18 of this report although it is not a requested response to a recommendation item. The Department believes it is important to explain the context of the information as it may not capture a comprehensive picture. GAO obtained the number from a pre-decisional/deliberative document where the Department was defining a range of possibilities for savings or costs. The cited data point came from a time when planning figures were still in flux and there was clearly double counting or lack of clarity of some requirements that resulted in this high figure. The DHA believes the number will be 14% and believes that the GAO did not have an opportunity to review more refined estimates since they were not available at the time of the study. Moreover, the Department believes there will be at least 10 percent reduction in MTF administration after the completion of the 702 consolidation.

In: Defense Health Care
Editor: Frederick Duncan
ISBN: 978-1-53615-175-6

Chapter 3

DEFENSE HEALTH CARE: ADDITIONAL ASSESSMENTS NEEDED TO BETTER ENSURE AN EFFICIENT TOTAL WORKFORCE*

United States Government Accountability Office

ABBREVIATIONS

ASD(HA)	Assistant Secretary of Defense for Health Affairs
DHA	Defense Health Agency
DOD	Department of Defense
FTE	full-time equivalent
KSA	Knowledge, Skills, and Abilities
MHS	Military Health System
MTF	military treatment facility

* This is an edited, reformatted and augmented version of United States Government Accountability Office; Report to Congressional Committees, Publication No. GAO-19-102, dated November 2018.

OASD(HA)	Office of the Assistant Secretary of Defense for Health Affairs
OPM	Office of Personnel Management
USD(P&R)	Under Secretary of Defense for Personnel and Readiness
VHA	Veterans Health Administration

WHY GAO DID THIS STUDY

The MHS includes more than 241,000 active duty, reserve, federal civilian, and contractor personnel who provide (1) operational medical care in support of war and other contingencies and (2) beneficiary medical care within DOD's hospitals and clinics.

The Senate Report 115-125 accompanying a bill for the National Defense Authorization Act for Fiscal Year 2018 contained a provision for GAO to review how DOD determines its mix of military, federal civilian, and contractor personnel. This chapter examines the military departments' planning processes for determining (1) operational medical personnel requirements, including an assessment of the mix of federal civilian, contractor, and active and reserve medical personnel; and (2) the most appropriate workforce mix at MTFs and any challenges in executing their desired workforce mix. GAO compared MHS staffing practices with DOD policy, and analyzed fiscal year 2017 budgetary data to determine the proportion of military, federal civilian, and contractor personnel. GAO also interviewed senior leaders at six MTFs.

WHAT GAO RECOMMENDS

GAO recommends that DOD, among other things, (1) assess the suitability of federal civilians and contractors to provide operational medical care; (2) develop full cost information for active and reserve component medical personnel; and (3) develop a strategic total workforce plan for the DHA to help ensure execution of an appropriate workforce mix at its MTFs. In commenting on a draft of this chapter, DOD concurred with each of GAO's recommendations.

What GAO Found

The military departments each have their own processes to determine their operational medical personnel requirements; however, their planning processes to meet those requirements do not consider the use of all medical personnel or the full cost of military personnel. Specifically:

- The Department of Defense (DOD) has not assessed the suitability of federal civilians and contractors to meet operational medical personnel requirements. Federal civilians and contractors play key roles in supporting essential missions, i.e., providing operational assistance via combat support. Military department officials expressed a preference for using military personnel and cited possible difficulties in securing federal civilian and contractor interest in such positions. An assessment of the suitability of federal civilians and contractors could provide options for meeting operational medical personnel requirements.
- When determining the balance of active and reserve component medical personnel, the military departments' processes generally do not consider full personnel costs, including education and benefits. Specifically, officials stated that the Army and the Navy do not consider personnel costs in their assessment of the appropriate balance between active and reserve personnel, and the Air Force's analysis had some limitations. DOD policy states that workforce decisions must be made with an awareness of the full costs. Further, in a 2013 report, DOD identified the cost of unit manning, training, and equipping as one of five factors that play a key role in decisions concerning the mix of active and reserve component forces. By

developing full cost information for active and reserve component medical personnel, DOD can better ensure an appropriate and cost-effective mix of personnel.

The military departments have taken actions, such as establishing policies and procedures, to assess the appropriate workforce mix for beneficiary care within Military Treatment Facilities (MTFs), but challenges remain. The military departments distribute military personnel across the MTFs and then use policies and procedures to consider risks, costs, and benefits to determine how to fill the remaining positions with federal civilians and contractors. However, a number of challenges, including lengthy hiring and contracting processes and federal civilian hiring freezes affect DOD's ability to use federal civilians and contractors. For example, senior officials at each of the six MTFs that GAO spoke with cited challenges with the federal civilian hiring process, and five of six MTFs cited challenges with the contracting process. As a result, senior officials from five of six MTFs reported discontinuing some services and referring patients to DOD's TRICARE network of private sector providers or Veterans Affairs facilities. The Military Health System (MHS) is also preparing for the phased transfer of administrative responsibility for MTFs to the Defense Health Agency (DHA), including management of the MTF workforce. According to GAO's report on agency reform efforts, strategic workforce planning should precede any staff realignments or downsizing. However, according to a senior official, the DHA has not developed a strategic workforce plan. Without developing such a plan, the DHA may continue to face the same challenges experienced by the military departments in executing an appropriate and efficient workforce mix at its MTFs.

November 27, 2018

The Honorable James Inhofe
Chairman

The Honorable Jack Reed
Ranking Member
Committee on Armed Services
United States Senate

The Honorable Mac Thornberry
Chairman

The Honorable Adam Smith
Ranking Member
Committee on Armed Services
House of Representatives

The Department of Defense's (DOD's) Military Health System (MHS) operates one of the largest and most complex health systems in the nation. DOD's total medical workforce of physicians, dentists, nurses, medics, and other health care providers includes active and reserve military personnel, federal civilian personnel, and private sector contractor personnel.[1] The MHS provides health care in two distinct settings: (1) operational medical care,[2] provided via deployable health care platforms such as forward surgical teams and combat support hospitals, in support of war, named or unnamed contingencies, and other operational missions; and (2) beneficiary medical care,[3] provided in DOD's military treatment facilities (MTFs), which

---

[1] In this report, we refer to the active and reserve military personnel, federal civilian personnel, and private sector contractor personnel working within the MHS as the total workforce. DOD's active components providing medical care include the Army, the Navy (which provides medical care for Marine Corps servicemembers and their beneficiaries), and the Air Force. The five reserve components providing medical care include the Army Reserve, the Army National Guard, the Navy Reserve, the Air Force Reserve, and the Air National Guard.

[2] For the purposes of this report, operational medical care and operational medical personnel requirements refer to health care provided via deployable health care platforms in support of war, named or unnamed contingencies, and other operational missions and the personnel who staff such platforms. In addition to providing health care to military servicemembers in and out of designated combat areas, DOD also provides medical care to communities in need as part of its humanitarian assistance and disaster relief services.

[3] For the purposes of this report, beneficiary medical care and military treatment facility (MTF) personnel requirements refers to health care provided in DOD MTFs and clinics in support of the medical readiness of military personnel and the general health of their dependents and other eligible beneficiaries and the personnel who staff such facilities.

include 51 military hospitals, 381 ambulatory care and occupational health clinics, and 247 dental clinics that serve to maintain the medical readiness of military personnel and the general health of their dependents and other eligible beneficiaries, such as retirees.[4]

DOD spends billions of dollars annually on its worldwide health care system.[5] Currently, health care costs constitute more than 8 percent of DOD's baseline budget request. For its fiscal year 2019 budget, according to DOD documentation, DOD requested $33.7 billion to fund the Defense Health Program, including the cost of health care activities, federal civilians, and contractor personnel, and an additional $8.9 billion in military personnel costs. The federal government's fiscal challenges, which we reported on in January 2017 and in other products, underscore the importance of DOD employing a strategic approach to determining the most appropriate and cost-effective mix of personnel to perform its mission.[6]

Senate Report 115-125, accompanying a bill for the National Defense Authorization Act for Fiscal Year 2018, included a provision for us to conduct a review of DOD's approach to assess and determine its workforce mix of active and reserve military personnel, federal civilians, and contractors within the MHS.[7] This chapter examines (1) to what extent the

---

[4] An MTF is established for the purpose of furnishing medical and/or dental care to eligible individuals. Statistics are projections for fiscal year 2018. Defense Health Agency, *Evaluation of the TRICARE: Program Fiscal Year 2018 Report to Congress; Access, Cost, and Quality Data through Fiscal Year 2017* (Feb. 28, 2018).

[5] DOD's fiscal year 2019 budget request of $50.6 billion for its Unified Medical Budget includes $33.7 billion for the Defense Health Program, $8.9 billion for military personnel, $0.4 billion for military construction, and $7.5 billion for health care accrual. The total excludes overseas contingency operations funds and other transfers.

[6] In January 2017, we reported on the nation's fiscal health and demonstrated that the federal government is highly leveraged in debt by historical norms and is on an unsustainable long-term fiscal path caused by a structural imbalance between revenue and spending. We concluded that addressing this imbalance would require significant changes in fiscal policy that will place budgetary strains on the federal government, including DOD, which accounts for approximately half of the federal government's discretionary spending. Discretionary spending refers to outlays from budget authority that are provided in and controlled by appropriation acts, in contrast to mandatory spending, such as that for Social Security, Medicare, or other entitlement programs, which is provided for in law other than appropriation acts. See GAO, *DOD: Actions Needed to Address Five Key Mission Challenges*, GAO-17-369 (Washington, D.C.: June 13, 2017) (citing to GAO, *The Nation's Fiscal Health: Action Is Needed to Address the Federal Government's Fiscal Future,* GAO-17-237SP (Washington, D.C.: Jan. 17, 2017)).

[7] S. Rep. No. 115-125, at 171 (2017).

military departments' planning processes for operational medical personnel requirements include an assessment of the mix of federal civilian, contractor, active and reserve medical personnel; and (2) the military departments' processes for determining the most appropriate workforce mix at MTFs and any challenges in executing an appropriate workforce mix as responsibility for MTFs' administration transfers to the Defense Health Agency (DHA).

For objective one, we compared military department efforts in planning for operational medical personnel requirements to DOD and department-level policies and guidance on workforce mix determination and identifying the full cost of personnel. Specifically, DOD Directive 1100.4 states that authorities should consider all available sources when determining workforce mix.[8] Moreover, DOD's 2017 Workforce Rationalization Plan recognizes DOD's federal civilians as an essential enabler of its mission capabilities and operational readiness, and DOD's National Defense Business Operations Plan for Fiscal Years 2018 to 2022 states that workforce rationalization strategies include, among other things, reassessing military manpower allocations for military essentiality and identifying functions and positions that are commercial in nature that may be appropriately or efficiently delivered via private sector support.[9] In addition, DOD Instruction 7041.04 has guidance for departments to identify the full cost of their active component, federal civilian, and contractor workforces, and in a 2013 report, DOD established five factors that play a key role in active and reserve component balance decisions, including the cost of unit manning, training, and equipping.[10] We interviewed officials from the military departments to discuss: (1) how they determine their operational medical requirements and if they identified the full cost of its active and reserve component medical personnel, and (2) the use of the active and reserve components for operational requirements and any efforts to assess the balance of active and reserve component medical personnel.

---

[8] Department of Defense Directive 1100.4, *Guidance for Manpower Management* (Feb. 12, 2005).

[9] Department of Defense, *DOD Workforce Rationalization Plan* (Dec. 12, 2017) and Department of Defense, *FY 2018-FY 2022 National Defense Business Operations Plan* (Apr. 9, 2018).

[10] Department of Defense Instruction 7041.04, *Estimating and Comparing the Full Costs of Civilian and Active Duty Military Manpower and Contract Support* (July 3, 2013).

To determine the extent to which federal civilians and contractors were deployed to provide medical care, we reviewed federal civilian and contractor deployment data from fiscal years 2013 through 2017.[11] To determine the mix of active and reserve component medical personnel, we analyzed authorization data from the Health Manpower and Personnel Data System for fiscal year 2017, which was the most recent year of data at the time of our review. To assess the reliability of both the federal civilian and contractor deployment data and the authorization data, we electronically tested the data to identify obvious problems with completeness or accuracy and interviewed knowledgeable agency officials about the data. We found the authorization data to be sufficiently reliable for the purposes described above. We found the deployment data to be limited in that it may not be sufficiently reliable for identifying the universe of deployments. However, we found the data to be sufficiently reliable for the purposes of reporting that federal civilians and contractors have been deployed to provide medical care. Finally, we interviewed officials from the Office of the Under Secretary of Defense for Personnel and Readiness (USD(P&R)), Office of the Assistant Secretary of Defense for Health Affairs (OASD(HA)), Defense Civilian Personnel Advisory Service, the military departments, selected combatant commands to identify considerations and any challenges of using different personnel categories as workforce alternatives for meeting operational medical requirements.

For objective two, we reviewed DOD and department-level policies and guidance on workforce mix determination and the departments' efforts in planning, staffing, and filling MTF requirements. To better understand policy and procedure implementation at MTFs we selected six MTFs — two each from the Army, Navy, and Air Force—to allow a cross-section of views concerning the management of the departments' workforce mix at the MTFs and hiring conditions in different types of labor markets. The two MTFs

[11] To determine whether federal civilians and contractors were deployed to provide medical care, we reviewed data from Defense Manpower Data Center. Specifically, to identify deployed federal civilians we used data from the Civilian Deployment System and to identify deployed contractors we reviewed data from the Synchronized Predeployment and Operational Tracker. These data may not be sufficiently reliable for identifying the universe of deployments.

from each department were selected based on consideration of average daily patient load and MTF bed size, which we obtained from the Defense Health Agency. For each MTF, we interviewed officials responsible for the leadership and management of MTF personnel and operations and requested and reviewed relevant documentation. We reviewed their responses, which highlighted some challenges related to achieving an appropriate workforce mix, and DOD's plans for addressing these challenges. We compared these to GAO's key questions to assess agency reform efforts, which note that strategic workforce planning should precede any staff realignments or downsizing.[12] We also reviewed how the planned transfer of administrative responsibility for MTFs from the military departments to the DHA might affect DOD management of military personnel within the MHS.[13] To identify (1) responsibilities of the military departments that may be transferred to the DHA, and (2) challenges that may continue under the new organizational structure, we reviewed relevant documentation and interviewed knowledgeable officials. We compared DOD's efforts to plan for these challenges to leading practices for results-oriented government, which state that cooperating federal agencies need to sustain and enhance their collaboration in several ways, including the development of policies and procedures to operate across agency boundaries and agreement on their respective roles and responsibilities.[14]

To determine the proportion of reported military, federal civilian, and contractor personnel providing or supporting care in MTFs, we obtained budgetary data for fiscal year 2017, which was the most recent full fiscal year of available data at the time of our review. To assess the reliability of these data, we compared it to the information reported in the fiscal year 2017

---

[12] GAO, *Government Reorganization: Key Questions to Assess Agency Reform Efforts*, GAO-18-427 (Washington, D.C.: June 13, 2018).

[13] The National Defense Authorization Act for Fiscal Year 2017 directed the transfer of administrative responsibility for MTFs from the military departments to the DHA. Specifically, the Director of the DHA shall be responsible for the administration of each MTF, including budgetary matters, information technology, health care administration and management, administrative policy and procedure, military medical construction, and any other matters the Secretary of Defense determines appropriate. Pub. L. No. 114-328, § 702(a) (2016) (codified as amended at 10 U.S.C. § 1073c).

[14] GAO, *Practices That Can Help Enhance and Sustain Collaboration among Federal Agencies*, GAO-06-15 (Washington, D.C.: Oct. 21, 2005).

Defense Health Program justification estimates published in February 2018 and interviewed knowledgeable agency officials about the data. We found the data to be sufficiently reliable for the purposes described above.

We conducted this performance audit from September 2017 to November 2018 in accordance with generally accepted government auditing standards. Those standards require that we plan and perform the audit to obtain sufficient, appropriate evidence to provide a reasonable basis for our findings and conclusions based on our audit objectives. We believe that the evidence obtained provides a reasonable basis for our findings and conclusions based on our audit objectives.

BACKGROUND

Composition of the MHS Total Workforce

The MHS has a dual mission of maintaining the skills of the medical force and providing health care and beneficiary medical care in its MTFs in the United States and overseas. It accomplishes this in part by providing (1) operational medical care via deployable health care platforms in an operational environment, such as forward surgical teams and combat support hospitals, and (2) beneficiary medical care in its MTFs in the United States and around the world. DOD's total workforce supporting this dual mission comprises three main components: military personnel (including active and reserve personnel), federal civilian personnel, and private sector contractor personnel. Active duty medical personnel simultaneously support operational medical care and the delivery of beneficiary health care to patients across the globe.

Reserve component medical personnel generally provide health care to deployed military personnel, but may also provide personnel to support MTFs when active duty personnel are deployed or otherwise unavailable. Federal civilians and contractors generally provide beneficiary care within MTFs. Figure 1 shows the number of the active and reserve components of

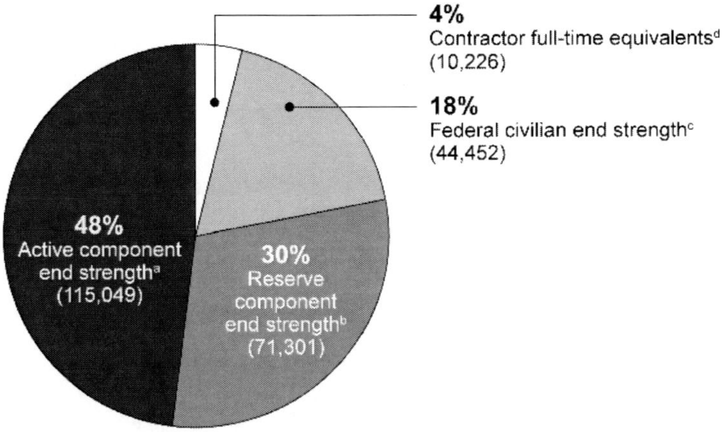

Source: GAO analysis of Department of Defense data. | GAO-19-102.

Note: This figure represents all military and federal civilian personnel with a primary medical occupation code and an estimated number of contractors providing medical services funded by the Defense Health Program in fiscal year 2017. This figure differs from figure 4 in this chapter in that figure 4 includes all personnel (i.e., medical and non-medical) supporting military treatment facilities.

[a]The active component end strength data are from GAO analysis of summary table A2 within the Health Manpower Personnel Data System report for fiscal year 2017. End strength represents the actual number of personnel on board at the end of the fiscal year.

[b]The reserve component end strength data are from GAO analysis of summary table R2 within the Health Manpower Personnel Data System report for fiscal year 2017. Reserve component end strength includes 65,123 Selected Reserve, 6,016 Individual Ready Reserve/Inactive National Guard, and 162 stand by reserves.

[c]The federal civilian end strength data are from GAO analysis of summary table C2 within the Health Manpower Personnel Data System report for fiscal year 2017. Federal civilian end strength includes only U.S. DOD Civilian Personnel and includes 43,809 full-time and 643 less than full-time federal civilian end strength.

[d]Contractor full-time equivalents were reported by the departments and represent the estimated number of contractor full-time equivalents servicing under medical care contracts funded by the Defense Health Program. According to a Defense Health Agency budget official, reported contractor full-time equivalents are estimates and cannot be validated. We have previously reported that a number of factors limit the accuracy and completeness of contractor full-time equivalent data. See, for example, GAO, *DOD Inventory of Contracted Services: Timely Decisions and Further Actions Needed to Address Long-Standing Issues*, GAO-17-17 (Washington, D.C.: Oct 31, 2016) and GAO, *Defense Acquisitions: Further Actions Needed to Improve Accountability for DOD's Inventory of Contracted Services*, GAO-12-357 (Washington, D.C.: Apr. 6, 2012).

Figure 1. Number and Percentage of the Department of Defense's (DOD's) Medical Military and Federal Civilian End Strength and Contracted Medical Services Full-Time Equivalents, Fiscal Year 2017.

the military, federal civilians, and estimated contractor full-time equivalents (FTEs) that comprised DOD's total medical workforce in fiscal year 2017.

DOD's Total Workforce Provides Operational Medical Care at Four Levels

DOD has established four levels of operational medical care provided to service-members and other eligible persons. The levels of care extend from the forward edge of the battle area to the United States, with each level providing progressively more intensive treatment.

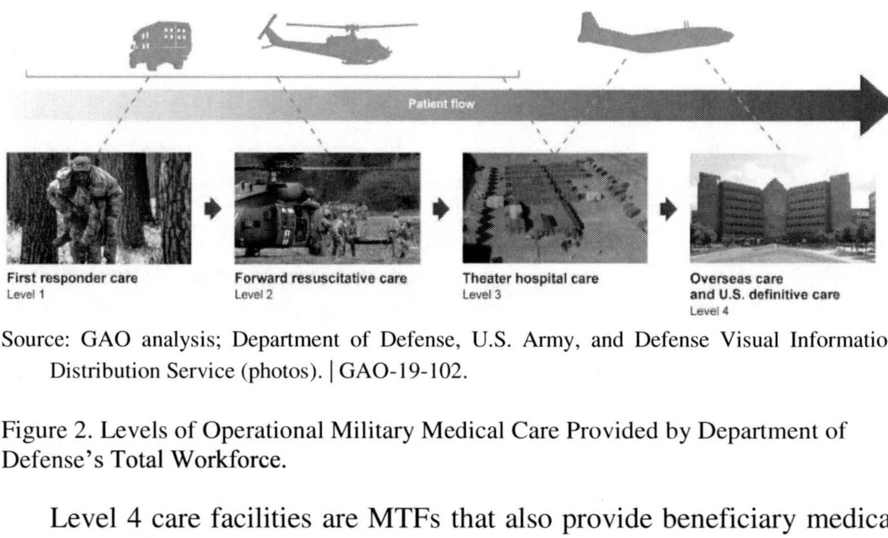

Source: GAO analysis; Department of Defense, U.S. Army, and Defense Visual Information Distribution Service (photos). | GAO-19-102.

Figure 2. Levels of Operational Military Medical Care Provided by Department of Defense's Total Workforce.

Level 4 care facilities are MTFs that also provide beneficiary medical care. In addition to the four levels of medical care, en-route care to transport patients is also provided via casualty evacuation, medical evacuation, and/or aeromedical evacuation from the point of patient injury, illness, or wounding.[15] Figure 2 illustrates the different levels of care.

[15] Casualty evacuation involves the unregulated movement of casualties aboard ships, land vehicles, or aircraft. Medical evacuation is the timely, efficient movement and en route care by medical personnel of the wounded, injured, or ill persons from the battlefield and/or other locations to and between MTFs. Aeromedical evacuation refers to the movement of patients under medical supervision to and between MTFs by air transportation.

The four levels of care are:

- Level 1—First responder care. This level provides immediate medical care and stabilization in preparation for evacuation to the next level, and treatment of common acute minor illnesses. Care can be provided by the wounded soldiers, medics or corpsmen, or battalion aid stations.
- Level 2—Forward resuscitative care. This level provides advanced emergency medical treatment as close to the point of injury as possible to attain stabilization of the patient. In addition, it can provide postsurgical inpatient services, such as critical care nursing and temporary holding. Examples of level 2 units include forward surgical teams, shock trauma platoons, area support medical companies, and combat stress control units.
- Level 3—Theater hospital care. This level provides the most advanced medical care available in Iraq and Afghanistan. Level 3 facilities provide significant preventative and curative health care. Examples include Army combat support hospitals, Air Force theater hospitals, and Navy expeditionary medical facilities.
- Level 4—U.S. and overseas definitive care. This level provides the full range of preventative, curative, acute, convalescent, restorative and rehabilitative care. Examples of level 4 facilities include MTFs such as Brooke Army Medical Center at Joint Base San Antonio, Texas and Naval Medical Center Portsmouth at Portsmouth, Virginia.

DOD Provides Beneficiary Medical Care in the United States and around the World

DOD's MHS workforce provides beneficiary medical care to 9.4 million eligible individuals, including active duty personnel and their dependents (i.e., spouse, children), medically eligible Reserve and National Guard personnel and their dependents, and retirees and their dependents and survivors. Located in the United States and around the world and ranging from small clinics to major hospitals, these facilities serve as training platforms for active duty medical personnel to maintain their skills and play a key role in the military departments' Graduate Medical Education programs for training medical professionals.

In addition to the direct provision of health care in its own hospitals and clinics, DOD maintains its TRICARE purchased care system that is used to augment the direct care system when needed. Through regional contracts, TRICARE administers the purchased care system, which comprises a civilian network of hospitals and providers.[16] Retirees who qualify for care under Department of Veterans Affairs' rules may also be eligible to receive health care within the Veterans Health Administration system of hospitals and clinics.

Legislation, Policies, and Processes Governing the MHS Workforce Mix

DOD's management of its workforce is governed by several workforce management statutes of title 10 of the United States Code, including:

- Section 129a directs the Secretary of Defense to establish policies and procedures for determining the most appropriate and cost-efficient mix of military, civilian, and contracted services to perform the mission of the department.
- Section 2463 directs the Under Secretary of Defense for Personnel and Readiness to devise and implement guidelines and procedures to ensure that consideration is given to using, on a regular basis,

---

[16] Prior to October 1, 2013, the TRICARE Management Activity, an entity within DOD, was responsible for overseeing DOD's regionally structured health care program. Upon its establishment, the DHA assumed management responsibility of numerous functions of DOD's medical health system, including the former TRICARE Management Activity.

DOD civilian employees to perform new functions and functions performed by contractors that could be performed by DOD civilian employees.

- Section 2461 directs that no DOD function performed by civilian employees may be converted, in whole or in part, to performance by a contractor unless the conversion is based on the results of a public–private competition that formally compares the cost of performance by civilian employees with the cost of contractors, among other considerations. There is currently a government-wide moratorium on performing such public-private competitions.

DOD's total workforce management policy generally emphasizes the need for agencies to utilize the least costly mix of personnel while ensuring the workforce is sufficiently sized, and comprised of the appropriate mix of personnel to carry out thc mission of DOD.[17] The departments use DOD guidance to assess the use of military, federal civilian, and contractor personnel, which includes the consideration of two key factors: (1) the risk to the military mission, and (2) the cost of the workforce. To help assess risk, the departments determine what work should be performed by military, federal civilian, or contractor personnel. For example, work that is inherently governmental[18] must be performed only by military or civilian personnel, while work that is commercial in nature could be performed by any personnel type.[19] To make this determination, DOD Instruction 1100.22 directs components to: use the manpower mix criteria outlined in the instruction to identify inherently governmental and commercial activities;

---

[17] DOD Directive 1100.4.

[18] An inherently governmental activity is a function so intimately related to the public interest as to require performance by federal government personnel. Pub. L. No. 105-270, § 5(2)(A) (1998). For example, operational control of combat, combat support and combat service support units; armed fighting or use of force deemed necessary for national defense; some aspects of security provided to protect resource and operations in hostile or volatile areas are inherently governmental activities.

[19] As defined in Office of Management and Budget (OMB) Circular A-76, a commercial activity is not so intimately related to the public interest as to mandate performance by government personnel. It is a recurring service that could be performed by the private sector and is resourced, performed, and controlled by the agency through performance by government personnel, a contract, or a fee-for-service agreement. OMB, Circular No. A76, *Performance of Commercial Activities* (May 23, 2003).

and review the annual inventory of commercial and inherently governmental activities.[20] In addition, DOD and the departments have established policies and procedures to assess the costs and benefits of different workforce mix options. DOD Instruction 1100.22 directs components to conduct a cost comparison of personnel when considering outsourcing[21] new requirements that are not required to be performed by government personnel, or when considering in-sourcing functions that are currently performed by private sector contractors.[22]

Roles and Responsibilities for Managing the MHS Workforce

Several officials have responsibility for governing DOD's management of its total workforce, including

- The Under Secretary of Defense for Personnel and Readiness (USD(P&R)). This official has overall responsibility for issuing guidance on total workforce management to be used by the DOD components, providing guidance on manpower levels of the components, and developing manpower mix criteria and other

---

[20] The annual inventory of commercial and inherently governmental activities is used to comply with reporting requirements set forth in statute and guidance, including requirements established by the Federal Activities Inventory Reform Act of 1998, Pub. L. No. 105-270 (1998), and in OMB Circular A-76.

[21] In the National Defense Authorization Act for Fiscal Year 2008, Congress enacted a moratorium on any study or competition relating to the possible conversion to performance by a contractor of any DOD function carried out at an MTF, until the submission of a certification and report by the Secretary of Defense. Pub. L. No. 110-181, § 1676 (2008). In 2009, Congress enacted both a DOD-specific and government-wide moratorium on public-private competitions regarding conversion to contractor performance of functions performed by federal employees. Pub. L. No. 111-8, § 737 (2009); Pub. L. No. 111-84, § 325 (2009).

[22] Department of Defense Instruction 1100.22, *Policy and Procedures for Determining Workforce Mix* (Apr. 12, 2010) (incorporating change 1, Dec. 1, 2017). DOD Instruction 1100.22 states that risk mitigation shall take precedence over cost savings when necessary to maintain appropriate control of Government operations and missions, or core capabilities and readiness. Furthermore, commercial activities shall be designated for civilian performance unless the private sector is the lower-cost provider or there is a legal, regulatory, or procedural impediment to using civilian personnel.

information to be used by the components to determine their workforce mix.

- The Under Secretary of Defense (Comptroller). This official is responsible for ensuring that the budget for DOD is consistent with the total workforce management policies and procedures.[23]
- The Secretaries of the military departments and heads of the defense agencies. These officials have overall responsibility for the requirements determination, planning, programming, and budgeting execution for total workforce management policies and procedures,[24] as well as having numerous responsibilities related to total workforce management as detailed in DOD guidance.[25]
- The Assistant Secretary of Defense for Health Affairs (ASD(HA)). This official serves as the principal advisor for all DOD health related policies, programs, and activities.[26] The ASD(HA) has the authority to: develop policies, conduct analyses, provide advice, and make recommendations to the USD(P&R), the Secretary of Defense, and others; issue guidance; and provide oversight to the DOD Components on matters pertaining to the MHS. Further, the ASD(HA) prepares and submits a DOD unified medical program budget which includes, among other things, the defense health program budget to provide resources for the DOD MHS.
- The Director of the Defense Health Agency (DHA). This official, among other things, manages the execution of policies issued by the ASD(HA) and manages and executes the Defense Health Program appropriation, which partially funds the MHS.[27]

---

[23] 10 U.S.C. § 129a(c)(4).

[24] 10 U.S.C. § 129a(c)(2).

[25] *See, e.g.*, DOD Directive 1100.4.

[26] Department of Defense Directive 5136.01, *Assistant Secretary of Defense for Health Affairs (ASD(HA))* (Sept. 30, 2013) (incorporating change 1, Aug. 10, 2017).

[27] In September 2013, the Defense Health Agency was established to support greater integration of clinical and business processes across the MHS.

Recent MHS Personnel Reform Efforts

The National Defense Authorization Act for Fiscal Year 2017 directed the transfer of administrative responsibility for MTFs from the military departments to the DHA. Specifically, the Director of the DHA shall be responsible for the administration of each MTF, including budgetary matters, information technology, health care administration and management, administrative policy and procedure, military medical construction, and any other matters the Secretary of Defense determines appropriate.[28] Since 2016, DHA's responsibilities in the administration of MTFs have been further articulated in DOD memoranda and in statute. In 2018, DOD directed that the DHA shall be responsible for: (1) the planning, programming, budgeting, and execution processes for the MTFs; (2) clinical and health delivery services in each MTF; and (3) for these services, the hiring and management of federal civilians and contract staffing.[29] Further, in 2018, Congress amended the law to specify that at each MTF, the Director of the DHA has the authority to determine total workforce requirements, direct joint manning, and address personnel staffing shortages, among other things.[30]

Also in December 2016, Congress enacted legislation that allows the prohibition of converting military medical and dental positions to federal civilian positions, which had been in place since 2008, to be lifted.[31] This change is contingent upon DOD satisfying a reporting requirement on the size and composition of its operational medical force. Specifically, Congress directed DOD to report on the process established to define the military medical and dental requirements necessary to meet operational medical force readiness requirements, and provide a list of those military medical and dental requirements.

---

[28] Pub. L. No. 114-328, § 702(a) (2016) (codified as amended at 10 U.S.C. § 1073c).

[29] Under Secretary of Defense for Personnel and Readiness Memorandum, *Authorities and Responsibilities of Military Treatment Facility Leaders, Service Leaders and the Military Medical Departments,* (Feb. 21, 2018). Under Secretary of Defense for Personnel and Readiness Memorandum, *Construct for Implementation of Section 702*, (May 22, 2018).

[30] Pub. L. No. 115-232, § 711 (2018) (codified at 10 U.S.C. § 1073c).

[31] Pub. L. No. 114-328, § 721 (2016).

Department Planning Processes for Operational Medical Personnel Requirements Do Not Include an Assessment of All Medical Personnel or the Full Cost of Military Personnel

The military departments each have their own process to determine their operational medical personnel requirements. After determining the number of medical personnel needed to support operational needs, the military departments generally consider only military personnel when conducting their planning processes to meet these requirements, and have not formally assessed the extent to which federal civilians and contractor personnel could be utilized. Further, the departments do not generally consider the full cost of active and reserve component medical personnel when determining their balance of active and reserve component medical personnel, and they have not developed such information to use in their assessment of active and reserve balance.[32]

Each Military Department Has Its Own Process to Plan for Operational Medical Personnel Requirements, Including the Balance of Active and Reserve Component Personnel

Each military department has its own process to plan for operational medical personnel requirements. The departments' operational medical personnel requirements are based on their analysis of DOD's Defense Planning Guidance and Defense Planning Scenarios.[33] Specifically, possible

---

[32] For purposes of this report we refer to the fully-burdened costs as full cost. The full cost of active duty military personnel includes, among other things, basic pay, special and incentive pays, allowances, permanent change of station, health and retirement benefits, education assistance, commissary benefits, and Veterans' benefits. For more information, see Department of Defense Instruction 7041.04, *Estimating and Comparing the Full Costs of Civilian and Active Duty Military Manpower and Contract Support* (July 3, 2013).

[33] The Defense Planning Guidance operationalizes the National Defense Strategy and provides guidance to the services on their use of approved scenarios, among other things, which serve as their starting point for making force structure decisions and assessing risk. These classified

casualty streams are estimated based on the scenarios, and the required medical support is determined in conjunction with department-specific medical planning factors, such as rotation policy, the population at risk, and evacuation policy, among others. Each military department incorporates these factors to estimate the number of medical personnel needed. The Army integrates medical planning into its general process for estimating all operational requirements, whereas the Navy and Air Force have separate, medical-specific processes. The following represents an overview of each military department's approach:

- Army. The Army uses its Total Army Analysis model to determine the number and type of support units across the Army, including medical forces, which will be needed to support the Army's combat forces in operational settings.
- Navy. The Navy uses a medical-specific model, called the Medical Manpower All Corps Requirements Estimator, to estimate its total medical personnel readiness requirements. The Navy readiness mission is to support all Navy and Marine Corps operational missions, including operational operations (such as hospital ships and expeditionary medical facilities) and day-to-day operations (such as ships, submarines, and Special Forces).
- Air Force. The Air Force uses a medical-specific sizing model named the Critical Operational Readiness Requirements tool to project its minimum military personnel requirements. This tool identifies the number of military medical personnel needed to meet requirements, including requirements for en-route casualty support, theater hospitals, and critical care air transport teams.

According to military department officials, the decision to apportion medical personnel requirements among the active and reserve components is based on an assessment of risk across a range of factors. In a 2013 DOD

---

scenarios are used to illustrate the missions articulated in the National Defense Strategy, including the need to defeat one regional adversary while deterring a second adversary in another region, homeland defense, and forward presence.

report issued in response to section 1080A of the National Defense Authorization Act for Fiscal Year 2012.[34] DOD noted that there are several important factors in active component and reserve component mix decisions, including, among others, the timing, duration, and skills required for anticipated missions.[35]

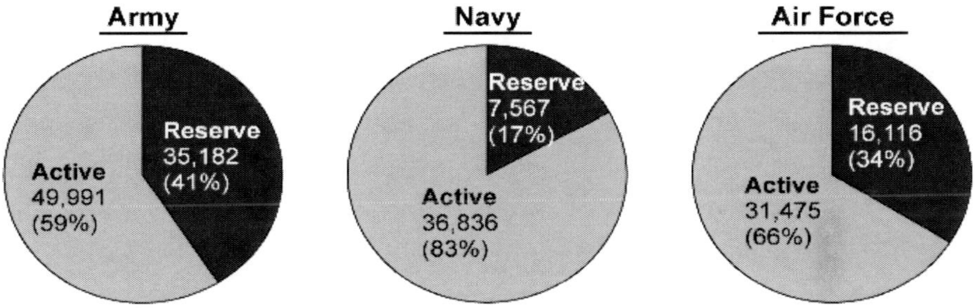

Source: GAO analysis of Department of Defense data. | GAO-19-102.

Note: Authorizations included in our analysis were reported in the Health Manpower Personnel Data System report for fiscal year 2017. Authorizations are for all medical personnel, regardless of funding. For our analysis of the reserve components, we analyzed authorization data for the Selected Reserve within the reserve components.

Figure 3. Number and Percentage of Uniformed Medical Personnel Authorizations by Component, Fiscal Year 2017.

Moreover, the report notes that active components are best suited for unpredictable and frequent deployments, dealing with complex operational environments, and unexpected contingencies and the reserve components are best suited for predictable and infrequent deployments. As noted in the report, active component personnel typically mobilize and deploy to theater the fastest. The sum of these considerations results in a different mix of active and reserve component medical personnel within each military department. Specifically, reserve personnel (as a percentage of the total workforce) varied by military department in fiscal year 2017, with reservists representing 41 percent of medical personnel of the Army, 17 percent of the Navy, and 34 percent of the Air Force, as shown in Figure 3.

[34] Pub. L. No. 112-81, § 1080A (2011).

[35] DOD, *Unit Cost and Readiness for the Active and Reserve Components of the Armed Forces* (December 2013).

DOD Has Not Assessed Using Federal Civilians or Contractors to Meet Operational Medical Personnel Requirements

The military departments have not assessed the extent to which federal civilians and contractor personnel can be used to meet identified operational medical personnel requirements. Specifically, after the military departments have determined their operational medical personnel requirements, they generally have designated all such positions as "military-essential" (i.e., the activity must be performed by a military servicemember) and have not formally assessed the extent to which civilians or contractors could be utilized to fill these positions, according to officials. Army, Navy, and Air Force officials stated that they have historically relied on active and reserve component military personnel when planning for operational medical requirements, with a few exceptions. For example, according to Navy officials, the few federal civilians that are planned to fill operational medical requirements are technical representatives who do not travel on ships for extended periods of time.

In interviews, military department officials cited key reasons for not incorporating federal civilians and contractors into their planning for operational medical care. Specifically, officials said they did not believe that federal civilians or contractors were viable workforce alternatives to military servicemembers for operational medical care roles and functions due to the unique nature of such assignments (e.g., providing medical care in a deployed setting). Moreover, officials noted that federal civilians and contractors supporting operational medical requirements are generally considered to be a temporary solution. Officials also expressed concern regarding their military department's ability to identify and recruit federal civilians and contractors for such positions. Officials stated that while there is currently no guidance outlining the potential role of federal civilians and contractors providing medical care in operational settings, they noted that DOD workforce mix guidance includes a provision that highlights the military-essential nature of medical personnel embedded in non-medical units engaged in hostile action.[36] However, this instruction does not otherwise address the role of federal civilians and contractors in providing medical care, including whether they can serve in medical-specific operational platforms, such as combat support hospitals providing level 3 care.

To ensure that its federal civilian employees will deploy to combat zones and perform operational roles such as critical combat support functions in theater, DOD established the emergency-essential civilian program in 1985. Under this program, DOD designates as "emergency-essential" those federal civilian employees whose positions are required to ensure the success of combat operations or the availability of combat-essential systems.[37] DOD's emergency-essential workforce is now governed under the Expeditionary Civilian Workforce program. DOD can deploy emergency-essential federal civilian employees either on a voluntary or involuntary basis to accomplish the DOD mission.[38] In certain DOD functional communities, federal civilians and contractors play a critical role in combat support roles. For example, as we previously reported, DOD relies on the federal civilian personnel it deploys to support a range of essential missions, including logistics support and maintenance, intelligence collection, criminal investigations, and weapons system acquisition and maintenance.[39] Further, as we have previously reported, DOD has long used contractors to provide

---

[36] DOD Instruction 1100.22.

[37] *See* 10 U.S.C. § 1508. DOD established the Civilian Expeditionary Workforce, which is now called the Expeditionary Civilian Workforce, in 2009 to create a cadre of federal civilians trained, cleared, and equipped to respond urgently to expeditionary requirements. Directive-Type Memorandum (DTM)-17-004 is the current guidance governing this workforce and states that it is DOD policy to identify and rely on a mix of capable military members and DOD federal civilians to meet global national security missions, and to include federal civilian employees in DOD's Global Force Management allocation process. Directive-Type Memorandum (DTM)-17-004, *Department of Defense Expeditionary Civilian Workforce* (Jan. 25, 2017) (incorporating change 1, effective Jan. 4, 2018).

[38] *See* DTM-17-004. Capability-based volunteers are employees who may be asked to volunteer for deployment.

[39] See GAO, *DOD Civilian Personnel: Medical Policies for Deployed DOD Federal Civilians and Associated Compensation for Those Deployed*, GAO-07-1235T (Washington, D.C.: Sept. 18, 2007) and GAO, *Human Capital: Improved Tracking and Additional Actions Needed to Ensure the Timely and Accurate Delivery of Compensation and Medical Benefits to Deployed Civilians*, GAO-09-1019T (Washington, D.C.: Sept. 16, 2009).

supplies and services to deployed forces.[40] Since the early 1990s, much of this support has come from logistics support contracts—contracts that are awarded prior to the beginning of contingencies and are available to support the troops as needed.

Although they are generally not a part of the military departments' planning processes, and there is no guidance dedicated to delineating the role of federal civilians and contractors in providing care in deployed operational settings according to officials, these personnel have deployed within the past 5 years. Based on our analysis of DOD federal civilian deployment data—for fiscal years 2013 through 2017—about 120 DOD federal civilians, including nurses, physicians, and technicians, were deployed to provide medical services. U.S. Central Command officials stated that they have used federal civilians minimally, and U.S. Africa Command officials stated they have not used federal civilians.[41] In addition, based on our analysis of DOD contractor deployment data for deployments from fiscal years 2013 through 2017, there were more than 1,900 deployed contractors providing medical services. U.S. Central Command officials told us that they have not used contractors to provide care to military personnel. Officials noted that the deployed contractors were not contracted by DOD for purposes of providing medical care and instead provided medical care to other contractors as they were part of a larger contract for other services, such as security services or logistics support.[42] U.S. Africa Command officials told us that they have used contractors to provide medical care to support casualty evacuation[43] and personnel recovery[44] requirements, which

[40] See GAO, *Military Operations, DOD's Extensive Use of Logistics Support Contracts Requires Strengthened Oversight*, GAO-04-854 (Washington, D.C.: July 19, 2004).

[41] For this review we selected two combatant commands (U.S. Central Command and U.S. Africa Command) in order to get their perspectives regarding workforce mix in theater. U.S. Central Command officials noted that individual services may have utilized federal civilians to provide care, a decision which would not have involved approval from their office.

[42] Responsibility for providing health services to contractors, whether it is the responsibility of the contractor or military, must be fully delineated in planning documents to ensure appropriate medical staffing. Joint Chiefs of Staff, Joint Pub. 4-02, *Joint Health Services* (Dec. 11, 2017).

[43] Casualty evacuation involves the unregulated movement of casualties aboard ships, land vehicles, or aircraft.

[44] Personnel recovery is the sum of military, diplomatic, and civil efforts to prepare for and execute the recovery and reintegration of isolated personnel.

includes providing medical care to military personnel and other eligible persons.

Officials with the Joint Staff Surgeon's Office and the Surgeon's offices at U.S. Central Command and U.S. Africa Command agreed with the possibility of using federal civilians and contractors for certain operational medical personnel requirements. Specifically, officials stated that federal civilians and contractors likely represent an acceptable workforce alternative if they are medically ready to deploy and appropriately trained for the unique environment at a fixed facility in theater, such as a level 3 fixed expeditionary medical facility or theater hospital.

While agreeing that the use of federal civilians and contractors for certain operational medical personnel requirements may be acceptable, officials also expressed concerns with this approach. A senior official with the U.S. Central Command Surgeon's office noted concerns regarding the pre-deployment training provided to contractors.[45] Specifically, the official stressed the importance of such training to operating effectively in the unique operational environment of a deployed medical team and that such training is only required to be completed by military personnel and DOD expeditionary civilians. U.S. Africa Command officials expressed concerns regarding challenges in obtaining clinical privileging rights (i.e., the right for a physician to perform specific health care services) for contractors supporting small teams in an operational setting. Further, OASD(HA) officials noted that a key factor to determining if federal civilians or contractors should be used to provide operational medical care is whether or not using those workforces would achieve any cost savings.

Moreover, officials with the Defense Civilian Personnel Advisory Service noted that they have had limited success with using DOD's Expeditionary Civilian Workforce program for the provision of medical administrative support and medical advising functions. A senior official from the U.S. Central Command Surgeon's office noted this was due to

---

[45] Military personnel and DOD expeditionary civilians complete pre-deployment training to receive tactical combat casualty care certification. The tactical combat casualty care course is intended to provide skills to assess and manage a combat casualty from point of injury to a higher level of care. Department of Defense Instruction 1322.24, *Medical Readiness Training (MRT)* (Mar. 16, 2018).

relatively few qualified federal civilians within the program with medical skills. Defense Civilian Personnel Advisory Service officials noted that the fiscal year 2019 force pool that defines the number and types of federal civilian requirements needed for the program included 7 medical related positions and none of these were for medical care; 1 was administrative and 6 were medical advisors. Defense Civilian Personnel Advisory Service officials stated that the DHA has a responsibility to build 1 or 2 of the medical advisor positions in the force pool into their planning as a continuing requirement, and noted that DHA has made some recent progress with 1 medical advisor scheduled to deploy in fiscal year 2019. While there may be challenges with utilizing federal civilian personnel to fulfill operational medical requirements, DOD also faces challenges with regard to military personnel. In 2018, we reported that DOD has experienced gaps between its military physician authorizations (i.e., funded positions) and end strengths (i.e., number of physicians), and that it did not have targeted and coordinated strategies to address key physician shortages.[46]

DOD has issued several documents to guide total workforce and personnel planning. DOD Directive 1100.4 states that authorities should consider all available sources when determining workforce mix, including federal civilians and contractors. Moreover, DOD's 2017 Workforce Rationalization Plan recognizes DOD's federal civilians as an essential enabler of its mission capabilities and operational readiness and noted that there are numerous opportunities for the military departments, combatant commands, and others to make well-reasoned adjustments to workforce mix. Further, DOD's National Defense Business Operations Plan for Fiscal Years 2018 to 2022 states that workforce rationalization strategies include, among other things, reassessing military manpower allocations for military essentiality, determining whether workload requires deployments and whether traditional military performance is necessary, and identifying functions and positions that are commercial in nature that may be appropriately or efficiently delivered via private sector support.

---

[46] GAO, *Military Personnel: Additional Actions Needed to Address Gaps in Military Physician Specialties,* GAO-18-77 (Washington, D.C.: Feb. 28, 2018).

Federal civilians and contractors are not incorporated into the military departments' planning to meet operational medical requirements because DOD has not performed an assessment of the suitability of federal civilian or contractor personnel to provide operational medical care. Such an assessment could assist in developing policy for use by medical planners in determining when, where, and how federal civilians or contractors may serve in operational roles. For example, an assessment may include what level(s) of care would be appropriate for federal civilians and contractors to support, if any, and factors to take into consideration in making such decisions, such as exposure to danger and cost. By conducting such an assessment and incorporating the results into relevant policies, DOD can have greater certainty that it is planning for the most appropriate and cost-effective mix of personnel to meet the mission, and, depending on the outcome of the assessment, more options to meet its operational medical personnel requirements.

The Military Departments Do Not Consider the Full Cost of Active and Reserve Component Medical Personnel When Planning for Operational Requirements and Do Not Have Full Cost Information

The military departments' planning to meet DOD's operational personnel requirements generally do not consider the full cost of active and reserve component personnel when determining the balance of active and reserve component medical forces. Officials from Army and Navy medical headquarters stated that cost generally does not inform their decisions about the balance of active and reserve personnel. Army officials noted they consider cost of a unit when making tradeoffs within the reserve component; however, cost was not cited by Army officials as a factor when determining between the active and reserve components. Navy officials noted that while it uses certain cost information when preparing the President's budget submission, cost is not explicitly considered when determining the balance of the active and reserve components. The Air Force is the only military department that has performed an assessment of the cost effectiveness of using active or reserve component medical personnel, although it had some limitations and did not impact the Air Force's active and reserve component mix decisions. Army, Navy, and Air Force officials cited other key factors which they consider in determining the balance of active and reserve component personnel, such as the availability of forces to deploy quickly, length of time needed in theater, capability needed, and frequency of deployments.

Moreover, the military departments have not developed full cost information of medical personnel to use in their assessment of active and reserve balance. Army and Navy officials stated that they do not maintain full cost information on its active component and reserve component medical personnel. Navy provided programming cost for the reserve component but these rates were averages across the reserve component and not specific to medical. The Air Force's 2016 High Velocity Analysis attempted to assess the cost of active and reserve medical personnel and identify potential efficiencies within its medical workforce. However, this study was limited because it did not include the full cost of active and reserve component medical personnel. Specifically, the Air Force analysis considered only compensation and did not consider other benefits, such as medical education costs, and used average pay for officers and enlisted personnel regardless of the specialty or skill level. However, the full costs for certain medical personnel, such as officers, are generally higher than average military pay, as they are eligible for a significant number of special pays and benefits, such as graduate medical education and training.[47] In fiscal year 2017, DOD obligated $788 million for special pays for active duty medical personnel, representing approximately 24 percent of the $3.3 billion obligated for all special pays across DOD, and $707 million for medical education. While the Air Force had full cost data for active component personnel, according to officials, they did not include it in their analysis because they did not have comparable cost data for the reserve

[47] DOD uses special pay programs as tools in its compensation system to help ensure that military pay is sufficient to field a high-quality, all-volunteer force, including those in hard-to-fill or critical specialties. Special pays are authorized in chapter 5 of title 37 of the U.S. Code.

component. Reserve medical personnel, when not mobilized, receive a fraction of what active duty personnel receive, and typically do not encumber significant education and training costs as reserve medical personnel generally are recruited as fully trained medical professionals.[48]

We have previously reported that when the reserve forces can successfully meet deployment and operational requirements, individual reserve-component units are generally less costly than similar active-component units.[49] However, the full cost of medical personnel can vary based on a number of factors. Specifically, more than one reserve-component unit may be needed to achieve the same output as a single active-component unit. For example, the Army has a policy that states reserve-component physicians, dentists, and nurse anesthetists shall not be deployed for longer than 90 days.[50] Thus, the Army would need to deploy four different reserve component physicians for successive 90-day rotations to fill a single 1-year active component requirement. Therefore, in some cases, using reserve units to achieve the same operational capacity over time may be more costly than using active units. However, the lack of full cost information on active and reserve component medical personnel is a barrier to an analytical-based determination on the balance between active and reserve component medical personnel.

In 2013, we reported limitations with the DOD-wide software tool developed by Cost Assessment and Program Evaluation—the Full Cost of

[48] Reserve component personnel may be eligible for special and incentive pays, including special pays for health professionals. Reservists are generally eligible for special and incentive pays during active duty training under the same conditions as active component personnel. Typically, they may receive a pro-rated portion of the full monthly amount corresponding to the number of days served. Reserve component members may also be eligible for special and incentive pays during inactive duty for training, and they typically receive such compensation at a rate proportional to the amount of inactive duty compensation they receive (i.e., one-thirtieth of the monthly rate for each unit training assembly).

[49] See GAO, *Active and Reserve Unit Costs: DOD Report to Congress Generally Addressed the Statutory Requirements but Lacks Detail*, GAO-14-711R (Washington, D.C.: July 31, 2014).

[50] Office of the Assistant Secretary for Manpower and Reserve Affairs Memorandum, *Army Medical Department (AMEDD) Reserve Component (RC) 90-Day "Boots-on-the-Ground" (BOG) Rotation Policy* (May 7, 2018).

Manpower—which, among other things, is used to identify the full cost of active duty military personnel.[51] Specifically, we reported that this tool has certain limitations for determining cost for certain cost elements. For example, instead of determining training cost by specialty, it estimates such costs by dividing total funding for such cost estimates by the number of military personnel. We recommended, among other things, that DOD, in order to improve its estimates and comparisons of the full cost of its workforces, develop guidance for cost elements that users have identified as challenging to calculate, such as general and administrative, overhead, advertising and recruiting, and training. DOD partially concurred with this recommendation but has not implemented this recommendation. We continue to believe that developing such costs is needed, especially for the medical community since training and education costs can be higher than in other communities. Moreover, in that report we also found that DOD did not include Reserve and National Guard personnel in their methodology for estimating and comparing the full cost to the taxpayer of work performed.[52] We recommended DOD, among other things, develop business rules for estimating the full cost of National Guard and Reserve personnel. DOD partially concurred with this recommendation but has not implemented the recommendation and noted that a cost estimating function for reserve component personnel would be more complex than for active component and DOD federal civilian cost estimates. While we agree that developing cost estimates for the reserve component could be more complex, we continue to believe it is advisable for DOD to implement our recommendation.

---

[51] GAO, *Human Capital: Opportunities Exist to Further Improve DOD's Methodology for Estimating the Costs of Its Workforces*, GAO-13-792 (Washington, D.C.: Sept. 25, 2013).

[52] GAO-13-792.

In a 2013 DOD report, DOD identified the cost of unit manning, training, and equipping as one of five factors that play a key role in decisions concerning the mix of active and reserve component forces.[53] According to the report, cost is often outweighed by other factors when making active component and reserve component mix decisions, but should always be considered in active component and reserve component mix decisions. Further, DOD policy states that workforce decisions must be made with an awareness of the full costs of personnel to DOD and more broadly to the federal government, and highlights that the full cost of active duty personnel extends beyond cash compensation, and also includes other costs such as education and training.[54]

The military departments do not assess the full cost of personnel when determining the balance of active and reserve component medical forces because there is no DOD requirement to do so. Although DOD guidance states that cost is one of several factors that should be considered in active and reserve component balance decisions, the military departments have not conducted assessments of the full cost of active and reserve component personnel to inform their decisionmaking. Further, DOD and the military departments are unable to conduct any such assessments because they have not developed full cost information for active and reserve component medical personnel. Without developing full cost information for active and reserve component medical personnel and using that information in its determinations regarding the correct balance of such personnel, decision makers will not have complete information to make cost-effective choices about the balance of active and reserve component medical personnel.

---

[53] DOD, *Unit Cost and Readiness for the Active and Reserve Components of the Armed Forces* (December 2013). The first three factors relate to the mission and include: sourcing for continuous operations (forward and homeland), surge and post-surge demands; mission predictability and frequency (force employment policy); and responsiveness of the force based on urgency of the task, unit integration, mission, or role. The fourth factor, retention and sustainment, adds stress on the force and should be considered, and the fifth factor, cost, is often outweighed by other factors when making active component and reserve component mix decisions, but should also be considered, according to the report.

[54] DOD Instruction 7041.04.

The Military Departments Have Established a Process to Assess the Appropriate Workforce Mix for Beneficiary Care within MTFs, but Face Challenges in Executing Their Plans

The military departments have taken actions, such as establishing policies and procedures, to aid the execution of the appropriate workforce mix for providing beneficiary health care within MTFs. However, the military departments face challenges in executing their plans in several areas, including lengthy hiring and contracting processes and uncompetitive salaries and compensation. Further, the transfer of administrative responsibility for MTFs from the military departments to the DHA may present challenges to the management of the military medical personnel.

The Military Departments Have Established Policies and Procedures to Evaluate the Risks, Costs, and Benefits of the Use of Personnel within Its Military Treatment Facilities

The military departments manage the workforce within their MTFs by using various policies and procedures to determine their workforce needs and help assess the risks, costs, and benefits of using military, federal civilian, and contractor personnel to carry out their missions. Currently, each military department is responsible for determining its MTF personnel requirements: that is, the number of personnel needed to operate its MTFs based on predicted demand for health care from their military and beneficiary populations. To determine MTF personnel requirements, the military departments use their respective suite of manpower models or standards based on a number of factors, including historical medical workload information and the size of population eligible for care. According to Army and Navy medical command officials, the Army and Navy suites of models respectively include at least 36 and 46 medical specialties, and generally express historical medical workload in relative value units, a metric of the level of professional time, skill, training and intensity to provide a given clinical service. In contrast, according to Air Force medical agency officials, the Air Force suite of standards includes 11 medical specialties and expresses workload in patient encounters.

According to military department officials, when considering how to meet their MTF personnel requirements given available resources, the number of military personnel is fixed and must be preserved since the operational medical personnel requirements support the readiness mission. The military departments therefore prioritize the distribution of military personnel across MTFs, and then consider how to fill the remaining authorizations with federal civilian personnel or by contracting medical services as appropriate. To make these decisions, the military departments utilize DOD workforce guidance, which requires a balance of risk and cost, but states that risk mitigation shall take precedence over cost-related concerns when necessary.[55] DOD total workforce policies and procedures are outlined in: (1) DOD Directive 1100.4, which establishes guidance for total workforce management; and (2) DOD Instruction 1100.22, which outlines policies and procedures for determining the appropriate mix of personnel. In 2018, we reported that a DOD study found that the cost of federal civilian and contractor full-time equivalents varied by organization, location, and function being performed.[56] According to Army, Navy, and Air Force officials, any changes to funded positions are made through formal processes and require an evaluation of the cost of the personnel options and the approval of the military departments' respective medical commands or agencies.

The military departments' collective decisions determine their workforce mix. Figure 4 shows the number and percentage of each personnel type that provided or supported care in DOD-owned and operated MTFs for fiscal year 2017, in the United States and overseas.

---

[55] DOD Instruction 1100.22.

[56] GAO, *Civilian and Contractor workforces: DOD's Cost Comparisons Addressed Most Report Elements but Excluded Some Costs,* GAO-18-399 (Washington, D.C.: Apr. 2018).

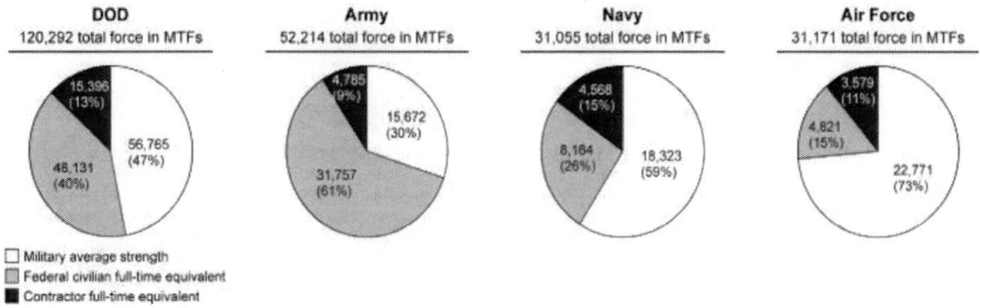

Source: Defense Health Program Operations and Maintenance, In-House Budget Activity Group data. | GAO-19-102.

Note: This figure represents all personnel (i.e., medical and non-medical) supporting in-house care in fiscal year 2017, which includes, among other things, military treatment facilities, medical center laboratories, and substance abuse programs. This figure differs from figure 1 in this chapter in that figure 1 includes all military and federal civilian personnel with a primary medical occupation code and an estimated number of contractors providing medical services. According to a DHA budget official, contractor full-time equivalents (FTEs) reported in the in-house budget activity group represent the estimated number of contractors supporting in-house care and cannot be validated. We have previously reported that a number of factors limit the accuracy and completeness of contractor FTE data, see, for example, GAO, *DOD Inventory of Contracted Services: Timely Decisions and Further Actions Needed to Address Long-Standing Issues*, GAO-17-17 (Washington, D.C.: Oct. 31, 2016) and GAO, *Defense Acquisitions: Further Actions Needed to Improve Accountability for DOD's Inventory of Contracted Services*, GAO-12-357 (Washington, D.C.: Apr. 6, 2012). The military average strength does not equal the total DOD due to rounding. The contractor and federal civilian total DOD force does not equal the sum of Army, Navy, and Air Force. The DOD total also includes 3,389 federal civilian FTEs and 2,464 contractors FTEs. These additional personnel are designated to provide services in the National Capital Region Medical Directorate and other DOD entities. Totals may not sum to one hundred percent due to rounding.

Figure 4. Number and Percentage of the Department of Defense's (DOD's) Total Workforce Providing and Supporting Care in Military Treatment Facilities (MTFs) by Personnel Type, Fiscal Year 2017.

Military Departments Face Challenges in Executing Workforce Mixes at Military Treatment Facilities, and DHA Does Not Plan to Develop a Strategy to Address These Challenges

The military departments face challenges to implementing their workforce mix of military, federal civilian, and contractor personnel. Our review, including interviews with military department officials responsible for medical personnel management and with the senior leadership of six MTFs, highlighted, as discussed below, the following distinct challenges: (1) the length of federal civilian hiring and contracting process, (2) uncompetitive federal civilian salaries and contractor compensation, and (3) FTE targets and hiring freezes.

Length of Federal Civilian Hiring and Contracting Process

Federal Civilian Hiring Process

Senior officials at each of the six MTFs we spoke with stated the federal civilian hiring process, including its length and restrictions imposed by statute or policy, impedes their ability to hire desirable federal civilian candidates. Officials primarily attributed delays to the extended time for human resources offices to post a position and to process and refer applicants for interviews. For federal civilian personnel in DOD medical locations in fiscal year 2018, DOD officials reported an average hiring time of: 121 days for the Army, 157 days for the Navy, and 134 days for the Air Force.[57]

Legal restrictions can also extend the hiring process and hinder hiring desirable federal civilian candidates. For example, senior officials at five of six MTFs cited a statute requiring a 180-day waiting period before retired military personnel can be hired as DOD federal civilians and noted valuable candidates with military-specific subject matter expertise will instead seek

---

[57] Defense Civilian Personnel Advisory Service officials provided this information, which depicts the average of the overall time-to-hire days for all hiring actions in DOD medical locations and includes medical occupations as well as other support occupations. According to officials, time-to-hire represents the initiation of the request for personnel action and ends with the entrance on duty, and medical locations represent locations where there are personnel supporting the medical community.

employment in the private sector.[58] Senior officials from one Air Force MTF stated they successfully submitted waivers to bypass the 180-day waiting period, but senior officials from one Army and one Navy MTF stated that the waiver process often takes as long as the waiting period.

Senior officials from each of the six MTFs stated that hiring authorities, such as direct or expedited hiring authority, can help address challenges, but officials at four of six MTFs also expressed concerns about the adequacy of such flexibilities. Direct-hire authority allows agencies to fill occupations that have a severe candidate shortage or a critical hiring need, and is meant to expedite hiring.[59] DOD designated a number of health care occupations as shortage category positions or critical need occupations in accordance with this expedited hiring authority.[60] In 2017, DOD reported that it used expedited hiring authority in approximately 30 percent of hiring actions for its medical employees.[61] Officials from one Navy MTF stated they have direct hiring authority, but their human resources office extends the process by requiring that the position be announced within the last 90 days, or else be re-announced, before they can utilize it. Army officials from one MTF stated interest in expanding the list of medical specialties granted direct hiring authority. Air Force officials from one MTF stated direct hire authority can help obtain qualified candidates, but does not necessarily shorten the hiring process.

Challenges in the federal hiring process are a longstanding issue. In 2003, we reported on the need to improve executive agencies' hiring process, with the majority of federal agencies included in our review reporting that it takes too long to hire quality employees.[62] Our 2016 review

---

[58] Section 3326 of title 5, U.S. Code, requires that 180 days pass before retired military personnel can move into a DOD federal civilian position, unless specific exceptions set forth in the statute apply.

[59] Direct hire authority was included in title XIII of the Homeland Security Act of 2002 and is codified in 5 U.S.C. § 3304(a)(3).

[60] Under Secretary of Defense for Personnel and Readiness Memorandum, *Extension of Expedited Hiring Authority for Shortage Category and/or Critical Need Health Care Occupations* (Dec. 14, 2015).

[61] DOD reported this was for the first three quarters of fiscal year 2017. Department of Defense, *Health Care Provider Appointment and Compensation Authorities: Fiscal Year 2017 Interim Report* (Washington, D.C.: Oct. 29, 2017).

[62] GAO, *Human Capital: Opportunities to Improve Executive Agencies' Hiring Processes*, GAO-03-450 (Washington, D.C.: May 30, 2003).

of the extent to which federal hiring authorities were meeting agency needs found that the Office of Personnel Management (OPM) and other agencies do not know if the authorities are meeting their intended purposes.[63] In 2018, we reported that DOD's review of selected sites, including two MTFs, found: varying use of hiring authorities, management unfamiliarity with all available authorities, and a belief among managers that expanded use of some authorities is needed to produce more quality hires.[64] Finally, our 2018 review of DOD laboratories' use of hiring authorities found that officials used hiring authorities, but identified challenges such as delays in processing the personnel action and the overall length of the hiring process.[65]

Contracting Process

Senior officials at five of six MTFs stated there are challenges in obtaining contractor services, including the process time before personnel are available to perform work and restrictions imposed by statute. Senior officials from two Air Force MTFs stated that after the contract is awarded, contractors may have up to 60 days to present a candidate; officials from one MTF stated if the MTF rejects the candidate, then the vendor has another 30 to 60 days to find a candidate. According to officials at one Air Force MTF, at times they have to consider whether to accept a subpar candidate or leave a position vacant. Further, senior Air Force officials stated that controls on contract spending limit their flexibility in hiring. To help fill temporary contract positions, which are less attractive to candidates, officials stated the Air Force pays higher rates to the vendor that include the salaries of the personnel and vendor's overhead costs. In 2018, we reported that DOD's negotiated price of a contract includes direct costs, such as labor and non-labor costs, and indirect costs, such as overhead, and service contractor profit.[66] Senior officials from the two Army MTFs stated that the moratorium on public-private competitions is a challenge because they

---

[63] GAO, *Federal Hiring: OPM Needs to Improve Management and Oversight of Hiring Authorities,* GAO-16-521 (Washington, D.C. August 2016).

[64] GAO-18-399.

[65] GAO, *DOD Personnel: Further Actions Needed to Strengthen Oversight and Coordination of Defense Laboratories' Hiring Efforts,* GAO-18-417 (Washington, D.C.; May 2018).

[66] GAO-18-399.

cannot outsource federal civilian functions to contracted services when there are shortages of military or federal civilian personnel, even when it is the optimal choice. For example, according to officials, contractors cannot perform the functions of a civilian position when a civilian position is vacated.

Uncompetitive Federal Civilian Salaries and Contractor Compensation

Federal Civilian Employee Salaries

Senior officials at each of the six MTFs stated it is a challenge to fill federal civilian medical positions because of lower salaries compared to the private sector. In 2017, DOD reported difficulty hiring and retaining health care workers due to competition from the private sector, among other things.[67] We have previously reported challenges related to the ability to provide competitive salaries for some DOD health care providers. Specifically, in 2015 we reported that officials from all three military departments stated their inability to create compensation packages for federal civilian mental health providers to compete with the private sector affected their recruiting and retention of providers.[68] In 2018, we noted similar concerns in recruiting military physicians.[69]

Senior officials from each of the six MTFs we spoke with stated that the ability to utilize hiring flexibilities, such as special salary rates, helps mitigate this challenge, but at four of six MTFs also expressed concerns about their adequacy. To provide higher pay for some occupations, OPM may establish a higher salary rate for an occupation or group of occupations in one or more geographic areas to address existing or likely significant handicaps in recruiting or retaining well-qualified employees.[70] Senior officials from four of six MTFs stated special salary rates are helpful but not

---

[67] Department of Defense. *Health Care Provider Appointment and Compensation Authorities: Fiscal Year 2016* (Washington, D.C.: Feb. 27, 2017).

[68] GAO, *Defense Health Care: Additional Information Needed About Mental Health Provider Staffing Needs,* GAO-15-184 (Washington, D.C.: January 2015).

[69] GAO-18-77.

[70] 5 U.S.C. § 5305; 5 C.F.R. §§ 530.301-323 (2018).

sufficient. Officials at one Navy MTF noted that two primary care providers left within the last year for better pay in the private sector, negatively affecting access to care. Officials at one Army MTF noted that the application for special salary rates can take 2 years or more, and therefore may not address short-term hiring needs. Further, officials from one Navy MTF stated they continue to face difficulty hiring for positions allowed special salary rates, such as pharmacist and registered nurse positions. Our 2017 review of federal agency use of special payment authorities approved by OPM—such as special salary rates—found that agencies reported that access to authorities had positive effects—such as on staff retention and applicant quality—but had few documented effectiveness assessments.[71]

DOD is also authorized to offer DOD health care personnel a number of salary rates established for Veterans Health Administration (VHA) personnel.[72] For example, DOD established a civilian physicians and dentists pay plan using this authority.[73] However, officials stated concerns about the rates' usefulness. Senior officials from one Air Force hospital noted that although the VHA salary levels are higher than the General Schedule levels that DOD typically offers, they may not be competitive with the private sector. Moreover, senior officials from one Army MTF expressed an interest in accessing VHA salary rates for additional occupations because Army personnel often leave to work at a nearby Veterans Affairs hospital for higher pay. In 2017, we reported on VHA physician recruitment and retention strategies and officials from the six VA medical centers in our

---

[71] GAO, *Federal Pay: Opportunities Exist to Enhance Strategic Use of Special Payments,* GAO-18-91 (Washington, D.C.: December 2017).

[72] OPM, under the authority of sections 1104 and 5371 of title 5, United States Code, authorized DOD to use certain personnel authorities for health care occupations under title 38, United States Code, chapter 74, subject to certain requirements and restrictions. *Delegation Agreement Between the Office of Personnel Management and the Department of Defense on the Use of Title 38 Authorities* (July 1, 2012).

[73] Department of Defense Instruction 1400.25, vol. 543, *DOD Civilian Personnel Management System: DOD Civilian Physicians and Dentists Pay Plan (PDPP)* (Feb. 12, 2018). In 2017, DOD reported that it had approximately 2,200 physicians and dentists under the PDPP. Department of Defense, *Health Care Provider Appointment and Compensation Authorities: Fiscal Year 2017 Interim Report* (Washington, D.C.: Oct. 29, 2017).

review stated that physician salaries were often below those offered by local private sector, academic, and some state government employers.[74]

Contractor Compensation

Senior officials from five of six MTFs stated private sector contractor vendors face the same challenges as the government regarding uncompetitive salaries. As a result, some contracts have low fill rates or go unfilled. For example, senior officials at one Navy MTF said one of its vendors has not been able to fill a clinical pharmacy position for more than a year. Additionally, senior officials at the other Navy MTF we spoke with stated that a vendor was not meeting its local needs because the fill rate at their MTF is lower than the average fill rate across all Navy MTFs, which is what the vendor is required to meet. Further, senior officials at two of six MTFs—one Navy and one Air Force—stated some of their vendors have attempted to fill positions by sending multiple providers on a part-time basis to fill the equivalent of one full-time position; they noted the part-time assignments are undesirable and can affect the quality of care.

FTE Targets and Hiring Freezes

Federal Civilian FTE Targets

Headquarters officials from each of the military departments stated that federal civilian FTE targets are a barrier to effective workforce mix management because they reduce flexibility in utilizing the most efficient personnel type to accomplish the beneficiary mission of the MHS. From fiscal years 2012 to 2017, OSD guidance directed the military departments to manage to a federal civilian FTE target.[75] These targets were intended to prevent an increase in the size of the federal civilian workforce, even when federal civilians' performance of work is most cost-effective. For example, Air Force headquarters officials stated that due to the federal civilian FTE

---

[74] GAO, *Veterans Health Administration: Better Data Evaluation Could Help Improve Physician Staffing, Recruitment, and Retention Strategies,* GAO-18-124 (Washington, D.C.: October 2017).

[75] According to senior DOD officials, this policy was prompted by DOD's efficiency initiatives first announced in 2010.

target, they generally default to hiring contractor personnel when new personnel needs arise. Further, Air Force headquarters officials stated they have not pursued in-sourcing of some contracted functions even though such actions might result in cost savings.

The federal civilian FTE targets had varying effects on the operations of the six MTF's we spoke with. Senior officials at two of six MTFs—one Navy and one Air Force—stated that they have not been adversely affected by the federal civilian FTE targets because the relatively high number of vacancies in their funded federal civilian positions means that they never exceed their target. Conversely, officials at one Air Force MTF stated they have considered hiring additional private sector contractor services when they reach their allowed federal civilian FTEs.

During the course of our review, DOD issued its National Defense Business Operations Plan for Fiscal Years 2018 to 2022, which states that it would discontinue the use of federal civilian FTE targets because they acted as artificial and arbitrary constraints on the workforce, and encouraged the military departments to utilize hiring flexibilities to identify the most appropriate and economical personnel type to achieve their mission.[76] In 2002 we reported that federal hiring policies should, among other things, avoid arbitrary full-time equivalent or other arbitrary numerical goals.[77]

Federal Civilian Hiring Freezes

Senior officials at five of six MTFs stated that federal civilian hiring freezes adversely affect MTF operations. As part of planning for sequestration in fiscal year 2013, DOD imposed hiring freezes on federal civilian personnel.[78] Further, there was a federal civilian hiring freeze from

---

[76] DOD. *FY18-FY22 National Defense Business Operations Plan* (Washington, D.C.: April 2018).

[77] GAO, *Commercial Activities Panel: Improving the Sourcing Decisions of the Federal Government*, GAO-02-847T (Washington, D.C.: September 2002).

[78] On March 1, 2013, pursuant to the Balanced Budget and Emergency Deficit Control Act of 1985, Pub. L. No. 99-177 (1985), as amended by the Budget Control Act of 2011, Pub. L. No. 112-25 (2011), the President ordered the sequestration of budgetary resources across the federal government. DOD's discretionary budget was reduced by about $37.2 billion, or about 7 percent in fiscal year 2013.

January 2017 to April 2017.[79] Senior officials from three of six MTFs reported that hiring freezes lower morale and elongate the already lengthy hiring process, even when they are granted waivers to continue to hire. Further, senior officials from one Army MTF stated hiring freezes limit their ability to shape their workforce, and often result in higher costs when they increase the size of their contracted workforce in accordance with their needs. We reported in 2018 that defense laboratory officials we surveyed identified government-wide hiring freezes as a challenge to hiring candidates, stating that candidates accepted other offers due to delays created by the freeze and that hiring efforts continue to be adversely affected even after a freeze is lifted.[80]

These three key hiring challenges limit the military departments' ability to strategically consider the advantages of converting one source of support to another, and limit their ability to hire the appropriate personnel type or for contract vendors to fill positions. According to senior MTF officials, these key hiring challenges and low fill rates in some areas can result in personnel gaps that can adversely affect the operations of MTFs. When personnel gaps arise, officials stated, military personnel often must work additional hours or must be borrowed from other facilities. Senior officials from one Navy MTF cited the example of a cost of about $16,000 in travel expenses for the temporary transfer of an active duty nurse stationed in Japan to work for a MTF in the United States for 3 months because the MTF was not able to fill the position by other means. Additionally, senior officials from one Air Force MTF noted that morale of its military staff is negatively affected by extra hours and additional responsibilities placed on them to ensure continued operations.

Further, officials stated that personnel gaps can negatively affect care. Due to concerns about patient safety, MTFs may decide to discontinue some services at MTFs. Senior officials from five of six MTFs reported discontinuing some services as a result of these challenges and referred

---

[79] *Presidential Memorandum on the Hiring Freeze*, 82 Fed. Reg. 8493 (Jan. 23, 2017); OMB, *Comprehensive Plan for Reforming the Federal Government and Reducing the Federal Civilian Workforce*, M-17-22 (Apr. 12, 2017).

[80] GAO-18-417.

patients to the TRICARE network or to Veterans Affairs facilities. Referring patients to the private sector can have secondary effects on MTF operations, such as on hospital accreditations. Senior officials from one Navy MTF noted that in the past fiscal year they had to refer patients to private sector care after two hematology-oncology physicians resigned, which may affect their hematology-oncology program's accreditation. Senior officials at the other Navy MTF stated that in the last fiscal year they could not meet the minimum staffing standards for labor and delivery staff and therefore sent patients to the TRICARE network. They noted they are also having difficulty filling key administrative positions related to quality control of laboratory services and are concerned about maintaining their pathology program accreditation.

Senior officials from MTFs reported varying fill rates for military and civilian personnel, and for the contractor personnel provided by private sector vendors.[81] However, officials from the MTFs we spoke with stated that fill rates may not illustrate the availability of personnel. For example, officials stated that authorizations for military personnel are counted as filled even when a servicemember is deployed and therefore not working at the MTF. In addition, MTF officials stated that any on-board civilians without corresponding authorizations inflate the civilian fill rate, resulting in a fill rate of greater than 100 percent. In addition, DOD officials noted that DOD pays for contracted services and does not directly employ contractor personnel. Therefore, the fill rate for contractors represents either the number of authorized FTEs in the individual contract or positions filled by contactors noted on the MTF's force planning document, which could also result in fill rates of greater than 100 percent, even as other positions remain unfilled. The MTFs that we spoke with reported the following fill rates:

- Two Navy MTFs. The fill rates for military personnel, federal civilian personnel, and funded positions designated for contracted services were 79 percent, 81 percent, and 94 percent, respectively,

---

[81] [8]We did not assess the reliability of the MTFs self-reported fill rate data. For military and federal civilian personnel, the fill rate represents the number of personnel on-hand (i.e., inventory) divided by the number of personnel authorized to work at the MTF.

at one Navy MTF[82] and 93 percent, 53 percent, and 62 percent, respectively, at the other MTF.[83]

- Two Air Force MTFs. The fill rates for military personnel, federal civilian personnel, and funded positions designated for contracted services were 98 percent, 86 percent, and 91 percent, respectively at one Air Force MTF[84] and 94 percent, 74 percent, and 90 percent, respectively at the other MTF.[85]
- Two Army MTFs. The fill rates for military personnel, federal civilian personnel, and funded positions designated for contracted services were 91 percent, 118 percent, and 87 percent, respectively at one Army MTF.[86] At the other MTF, the fill rate for military personnel fill rate was 94 percent and for federal civilian personnel was 107 percent, but the MTF officials did not provide fill rate information for positions designated for contracted services because there are no corresponding authorizations on their force planning document.[87]

DOD has been taking some steps to attempt to address these key hiring challenges. Specifically, DOD's 2016 Strategic Workforce Plan included steps DOD was taking to address personnel gaps, such as a targeted

[82] According to officials, data are as of July 2018, and military personnel information includes active duty members only, information for health care providers and nurses only, and contractor authorizations represent authorizations documented on the activity manpower document.

[83] According to officials, data represent fiscal year 2018, military personnel information includes active duty members only, and contractor authorizations represent FTEs authorized on each contract.

[84] According to officials, data represent fiscal year 2017 and include 9 federal civilian over hires or overages. Further, officials stated that contractor authorizations represent FTEs authorized on each contract.

[85] According to officials, data represent fiscal year 2018, and generally exclude residents, students, federal civilian over hires, and contracts funded outside of the normal budgeting process. Further, officials stated that contractor authorizations represent FTEs authorized during the budgeting process.

[86] According to officials, data represent fiscal year 2018, 10 military personnel are in training positions that do not have corresponding authorizations, and contractor authorizations represent FTEs authorized on each contract.

[87] According to officials, data represent fiscal year 2018 and the federal civilian fill rate is over 100 percent because it includes 235 federal civilian over hires that do not have a corresponding authorization on the force planning document.

recruitment program for critical skills, including 27 harder-to-fill medical occupations. In 2018, DOD published a Human Capital Operating Plan which states that it replaces the previously required Strategic Workforce Plan, but DOD does not yet have a plan of action specific to the medical professions.[88] Further, DOD officials stated that components are encouraged to consider developing their own human capital operating plans. With regard to contracting, in response to a requirement in the National Defense Authorization Act for Fiscal Year 2017, DOD issued a status report in January 2018 on the development of its acquisition strategy for health care services at MTFs.[89] The report notes that contracting for health care services is fragmented, and the report outlines DOD's plan to move toward a single contract vehicle for health care services and to establish metrics for the strategy, such as measurement of contract fill rates.[90]

While these steps represent efforts to address these challenges, responsibility for management of the federal civilian and contractor workforces within the MHS will soon see significant changes. Specifically, in December 2016, Congress directed the transfer of administrative responsibility for MTFs from the military departments to the DHA.[91] Further, Congress amended the law in 2018 to specify that the transfer should be completed by September 30, 2021.[92] The law also states that at each MTF, the Director of the DHA has the authority to determine total workforce requirements, direct joint manning, and address personnel staffing shortages, among other things.

Although the DHA will soon begin to assume these responsibilities and the challenges associated with them, a senior OASD(HA) official responsible for human capital issues stated that the DHA currently has no

[88] The Human Capital Operating Plan supports the National Defense Business Operations Plan—a supplement to the National Defense Strategy—and is part of an ongoing DOD effort to align and implement human capital strategy with overall performance strategy. Effective April 11, 2017, OPM updated 5 C.F.R. § 250 subpart B to replace the previously required strategic human capital plan and DOD Strategic Workforce Plan with the Human Capital Operating Plan.

[89] Pub. L. No. 114-328, § 727 (2016).

[90] DOD, *Report on Section 727 of the National Defense Authorization Act for Fiscal Year 2017 (Public Law 114-328)* (Washington, D.C.: Jan. 11, 2018).

[91] Pub. L. No. 114-328, § 702 (2016) (codified as amended at 10 U.S.C. § 1073c).

[92] Pub. L. No. 115-232, § 711 (2018) (codified at 10 U.S.C. § 1073c).

strategic total workforce plan, or similar document, to help ensure execution of an appropriate workforce mix at its MTFs. According to GAO's key questions to assess agency reform efforts, strategic workforce planning should precede any staff realignments or downsizing, so that changed staff levels do not inadvertently produce skills gaps or other adverse effects that could result in increased use of overtime and contracting.[93] GAO's key principles for effective strategic workforce planning and applicable federal regulations have shown that addressing a critical human capital challenge—such as closing or reducing personnel gaps—requires tailored human capital strategies and tools and metrics by which to monitor and evaluate progress toward reducing gaps.[94] Although many hiring challenges are longstanding government-wide issues, GAO's model of strategic human capital management states that agencies need not wait for comprehensive civil service reform to modernize their human capital approaches.[95] In addition, according to OPM's standards for strategic workforce planning, human capital strategies should be integrated with acquisition plans, among other things, such as DOD's acquisition strategy for health care services at MTFs.[96]

As the DHA finalizes its plans for assuming administrative control of MTFs, senior leaders may find that they face the same challenges reported by the military departments in executing an appropriate workforce mix. DHA could mitigate these challenges to executing the appropriate workforce mix in the MTFs by engaging in strategic workforce planning, including tailored human capital strategies, tools, and metrics by which to monitor and evaluate progress toward reducing gaps, and integrating this planning with DOD's acquisition strategy for health care services at MTFs.

---

[93] GAO, *Government Reorganization: Key Questions to Assess Agency Reform Efforts*, GAO-18-427 (Washington, D.C.: June 13, 2018).

[94] GAO-04-39; and 5 C.F.R. § 250.204 (2018).

[95] GAO, *A Model of Strategic Human Capital Management*, GAO-02-373SP (Washington, D.C.: Mar. 15, 2002).

[96] 5 C.F.R. § 250.203 (2018).

The Military Departments and DHA Have Not Decided How Military Personnel Will Meet Operational and Beneficiary Missions after the Transfer of Administrative Responsibility for MTFs to DHA

The planned transfer of administrative responsibility for MTFs from the military departments to the DHA may present challenges to DOD's management of military personnel. Specifically, the military departments and DHA have not determined how military personnel will meet both the operational and beneficiary missions of the MHS after the transfer of administrative responsibility for MTFs to the DHA. Historically, each military department has been responsible for managing its military personnel to ensure it meets its operational mission and appropriately staffs its MTFs, and the challenge of balancing these missions was the responsibility of each respective military department. However, the transfer of administrative responsibility for MTFs to the DHA will separate these missions—the operational mission will be the responsibility of the military departments, and the beneficiary mission will be the responsibility of the DHA, with military personnel used to support both missions. The plan for transfer of administrative responsibility for MTFs to the DHA states that the military departments will retain ultimate control over military personnel, who will work within the MTFs on a day-to-day basis to maintain their readiness to provide operational medical care, while the DHA will eventually assume responsibility for federal civilian and contractor personnel and all other aspects of MTF management.[97] DOD officials stated that the planned transfer will allow the military departments to focus their attention on readiness to provide operational medical care, while the DHA will focus its attention on efficient management of beneficiary health care operations.[98] As a result of this separation of missions, challenges in the management of military personnel could be exacerbated by transfer of responsibility for

---

[97] DOD, *Final Plan to Implement 1073c of Title 10, United States Code Final Report,* (June 30, 2018).

[98] *Final Plan to Implement 1073c of Title 10, United States Code Final Report.*

achieving these missions to separate organizations in the following three ways.

First, DHA and the military departments have not clearly identified how they will manage the assignment of military personnel to MTFs. The implementation plan for transfer of administrative responsibility for MTFs to the DHA states that the departments will continue to be responsible for assignment of military personnel to MTFs. However, DOD's stated desire to place greater emphasis on the readiness mission may affect current MTF staffing practices. For example, military department officials told us that it is common practice to assign military personnel to locations that face challenges in hiring federal civilian and contractor medical personnel to maintain access to medical care in these locations. However, the transfer implementation plan states that the departments will provide military personnel to the MTFs only to the extent that the MTFs can provide sufficient workload to maintain providers' military medical Knowledge, Skills, and Abilities (KSAs). KSAs are a metric for military operational readiness that DOD has not yet finalized. Officials responsible for planning the transfer of administrative responsibility for MTFs to the DHA stated that the emphasis on fulfilling KSAs in the future may result in concentrating military providers in larger MTFs, which can provide opportunities for providers to fulfill KSAs. However, this change could create a disadvantage for smaller facilities, which may not be able to provide military providers with as much practice and already face challenges in hiring federal civilian and contractor personnel.

Second, DHA and the military departments have not clearly identified how they will mitigate the effect of deployments of military medical personnel on MTF operations. When medical personnel are deployed out of MTFs to provide operational care, their absence can create a gap or reduction in capability at the affected MTF, according to military department officials. The military departments, prior to the transfer, manage deployments and are responsible for ensuring appropriate staffing at the MTFs in the absence of deployed personnel. Officials at all six of the MTFs we visited cited challenges with mitigating the effect of deployments on MTF operations. DOD has stated that after the transition, there will be no barriers to the military departments' access to personnel for deployment, and has highlighted options for addressing staffing gaps, such as using borrowed military personnel, contractors, or referral to the TRICARE network. However, officials at all six of the MTFs we spoke with stated that contracting for medical services was not sufficiently timely or effective, and officials at one MTF noted that referral to the TRICARE network was difficult in their area.

According to officials within the MTFs of the National Capital Region, which is directly managed by the DHA and not the military departments, management of deployments and their adverse effect on hospital staffing has been a challenge. For example, officials cited a period in the summer of 2017 when, due to overlapping deployments across military departments, 8 of 9 general surgeons at Fort Belvoir Community Hospital in Virginia were simultaneously deployed, and patients had to be referred to private providers within the TRICARE network or sent to Walter Reed National Military Medical Center in Maryland.

Although the military departments and the DHA have executed a Memorandum of Agreement concerning coordination for service personnel to fill scheduled deployments, this does not always prevent gaps in medical specialties. For example, officials noted that requests for volunteer deployments are not always vetted through NCR management. Further, addressing these gaps can be challenging. Specifically, officials cited difficulties in successfully contracting for medical services and reported that requests for backfill support from the reserve components has associated costs and is difficult to execute.

Third, DHA and the military departments have not clearly identified how they will manage changes to the size or composition of the active duty medical workforce that affect workforce balance within MTFs. Since 2008, the military departments have been prohibited from converting medical positions designated for military personnel to positions that can be filled by federal civilians—even when such conversions would result in cost savings.[99] Air Force headquarters officials noted that they have identified

---

[99] Pub. L. No. 110-181, § 721 (2008).

more than 4,000 medical positions to review for possible conversion to achieve cost savings, particularly in medical specialties with excess military personnel, such as family practice and pharmacy. Air Force officials previously identified 4,724 positions for conversion beginning in fiscal year 2005, of which 1,449 were completed before the prohibition was enacted. The Army planned to convert 4,340 military positions from fiscal year 2006 through fiscal year 2011, of which 1,459 were completed before the prohibition was enacted. The Army restored 165 of planned conversions for fiscal year 2007, and reversed, or offset the remaining through growth in the active duty medical force after the prohibition was enacted.

The National Defense Authorization Act for Fiscal Year 2017 allows for the prohibition on such conversions to be lifted after DOD submits a report that defines the military medical and dental requirements necessary to meet operational medical force readiness requirements, and lists the positions necessary to meet such requirements.[100] However, decisions on conversions taken by the departments could affect MTF operations. Specifically, existing challenges with hiring federal civilian personnel could create challenges with military-to-civilian conversions. For example, DOD has stated that during the previous round of military to federal civilian conversions, changes in local market conditions affected the ability of the military departments to fill converted positions with civilians in a timely fashion.[101] Medical headquarters officials the Army stated that they currently have no intention to use conversions if the prohibition is lifted; Navy officials stated they currently do not plan to use conversions since their military personnel requirements exceed their authorizations. Senior officials from one Navy MTF we spoke with stated that if conversions occurred, recruitment and retention challenges related to hiring federal civilian employees would need to be addressed to ensure such positions are filled.

In addition, military department policies can affect workforce balance within MTFs. Specifically, in its modeling for operational medical personnel requirements, the Air Force includes a preference for uniformed personnel to receive primary care from uniformed medical personnel. Officials told us

---

[100] Pub. L. No. 114-328, § 721 (2016).

[101] DOD, *Military Health System Modernization Study Team Report* (May 29, 2015).

that this approach, known as the Critical Home Station, is because Air Force leadership believes that performance of this function by military personnel provides for increased accountability for medical readiness. For example, senior officials from one Air Force MTF stated they believe the policy is important for the Air Force to maintain access to information about health factors that could render a servicemember not medically qualified to deploy. Air Force medical headquarters officials estimate that the policy results in 2,000 positons reserved for military personnel that could be designated for federal civilian or contractor performance.

Leading practices for results-oriented government state that cooperating federal agencies need to sustain and enhance their collaboration in several ways, including the development of policies and procedures to operate across agency boundaries and agreement on their respective roles and responsibilities.[102] However, planning for the transition by the DHA and the military departments has not yet included development of policies and procedures for management of military personnel and agreement on specific roles and responsibilities for the military departments and the DHA in this process. The MHS process for collaborating across agency boundaries, known as MHS Governance, emphasizes collaborative work in the management of the MHS. This forum could provide an opportunity for the military departments and the DHA to develop policies and procedures for management of military personnel and agree on specific roles and responsibilities for the military departments and the DHA in this process. Until DHA and the military departments develop such policies and procedures and agrees on roles and responsibilities, the MHS may continue to face a number of challenges related to the transfer of administrative responsibility for MTFs to the DHA.

---

[102] GAO, *Practices That Can Help Enhance and Sustain Collaboration among Federal Agencies*, GAO-06-15 (Washington, D.C.: Oct. 21, 2005).

Conclusion

Given the size of the MHS, its central importance to the success of DOD's mission, and its cost, having the right mix of military, federal civilian, and contractor personnel providing medical care within MTFs and in deployed operational settings should be a key priority for DOD leadership. While the military departments have policies and procedures in place to assess medical workforce mix in both settings, the shortcomings we have highlighted present barriers to achieving an appropriate workforce mix. Recently, such as in the 2018 National Defense Business Operations Plan, DOD has emphasized the need to reassess who can most efficiently perform all aspects of DOD's mission. However, the military departments' planning processes for operational medical personnel requirements continue to rely solely on military personnel, despite the use of federal civilians and contractors in operational settings, and the military departments have not developed full information on the cost of their medical forces and incorporated such information into decision-making processes about the mix of active and reserve component personnel. Similarly, the transfer of administrative responsibility for MTFs to the DHA represents an opportunity to reassess workforce mix at the MTFs. However, long-standing challenges in the management of federal civilian and contractor personnel, coupled with challenges related to the management of medical personnel after the transfer, could overshadow and cast doubt on the success of that reform. Without addressing the concerns we have highlighted, DOD may miss the opportunity presented by current transformation efforts in the MHS to ensure it has in place the most cost-effective mix of personnel in its workforce to accomplish its medical mission.

Recommendations for Executive Action

We are making five recommendations to the Department of Defense.

1. The Secretary of Defense should ensure that the Assistant Secretary of Defense for Health Affairs, in coordination with the military departments, perform an assessment of the suitability of federal civilian and contractor personnel to provide operational medical care and incorporate the results of the assessment into relevant policies, if warranted. (Recommendation 1)
2. The Secretary of Defense should ensure that the Under Secretary of Defense for Personnel and Readiness require consideration of cost when making determinations regarding the mix of active and reserve component medical personnel. (Recommendation 2)
3. The Secretary of Defense should ensure that the Assistant Secretary of Defense for Health Affairs, in collaboration with the Director of Cost Assessment and Program Evaluation and the military departments, develop full cost information for active and reserve component medical personnel, and the military departments use that information in its determinations regarding the mix of active and reserve component medical personnel. (Recommendation 3)
4. The Secretary of Defense should ensure that the Director of the Defense Health Agency develop a strategic total workforce plan which includes, among other things: (1) tailored human capital strategies, tools, and metrics by which to monitor and evaluate progress toward reducing personnel gaps, and; (2) integration of human capital strategies with acquisition plans, such as DOD's acquisition strategy for health care services at DOD's military treatment facilities. (Recommendation 4)
5. The Secretary of Defense and the Secretaries of the Army, the Navy, and the Air Force, respectively, should ensure that accompanying the transfer of administrative responsibility for military treatment facilities to the Defense Health Agency, that the Defense Health Agency and the military departments develop policies and procedures for management of military personnel, including agreement on specific roles and responsibilities for the military departments and the Defense Health Agency in this process. (Recommendation 5)

AGENCY COMMENTS

In written comments on a draft of this chapter, DOD concurred with our five recommendations concerning additional assessments needed to better ensure an efficient MHS total workforce. DOD's comments are reprinted in appendix II.

Brenda S. Farrell
Director
Defense Capabilities and Management

APPENDIX I: SCOPE AND METHODOLOGY

To address the extent to which the military departments' planning process for operational medical personnel requirements have assessed the mix of federal civilian, contractor, active and reserve medical personnel (i.e., workforce mix), we compared the military departments' efforts in planning for operational medical personnel requirements to the Department of Defense (DOD) and department-level policies and guidance on workforce mix determination and identifying the full cost of its military medical personnel. DOD Directive 1100.4 states that authorities should consider all available sources when determining workforce mix.[103] DOD Instruction 1100.22 directs the steps that workforce planning authorities must take in planning for personnel requirements and emphasizes consideration of all potential workforce sources and an accurate understanding of personnel costs.[104] We also reviewed related DOD documentation on identifying military essential positons and the use of alternative workforces.

---

[103] Department of Defense Directive 1100.4, *Guidance for Manpower Management* (Feb. 12, 2005).

[104] Department of Defense Instruction 1100.22, *Policy and Procedures for Determining Workforce Mix* (Apr. 12, 2010) (incorporating change 1 Dec. 1 2017).

Specifically, DOD's National Defense Business Operations Plan for fiscal years 2018 through 2022 states that workforce rationalization strategies include, among other things, reassessing military manpower allocations for military essentiality and identifying functions and positions that are commercial in nature that may be appropriately or efficiently delivered via private sector support.[105] Moreover, DOD's 2017 Workforce Rationalization Plan recognizes DOD's civilians as an essential enabler of its mission capabilities and operational readiness and noted that there are numerous opportunities for the military departments, combatant commands, and others to make well-reasoned adjustments to workforce mix.[106]

To determine the extent to which federal civilians and contractors were deployed to provide medical care we reviewed federal civilian and contractor deployment data from fiscal years 2013 through 2017.[107] We analyzed data for this timeframe to enable us to identify deployments over the last 5 years, and fiscal year 2017 was the most recent full fiscal year of available data at the time of our review. To assess the reliability of these data, we electronically tested the data to identify obvious problems with completeness or accuracy and interviewed knowledgeable agency officials about the data. We found the data to be limited in that the deployment data may not be sufficiently reliable for identifying the universe of deployments. However, we found the data to be sufficiently reliable for the purposes of reporting that federal civilians and contractors have been deployed to provide medical care. Further, we interviewed officials from the Office of the Under Secretary of Defense for Personnel and Readiness (USD(P&R)), Office of the Assistant Secretary of Defense for Health Affairs

[105] Department of Defense, *FY 2018-FY 2022 National Defense Business Operations Plan* (Apr. 9, 2018).

[106] Department of Defense, *DOD Workforce Rationalization Plan* (Dec. 12, 2017).

[107] To determine whether federal civilians and contractors were deployed to provide medical care, we reviewed data from the Defense Manpower Data Center. Specifically, to identify deployed federal civilians we used data from the Civilian Deployment System and to identify deployed contractors we reviewed data from the Synchronized Predeployment and Operational Tracker. These data may not be sufficiently reliable for identifying the universe of deployments.

(OASD(HA)), Defense Civilian Personnel Advisory Service, the military departments, and selected combatant commands to identify considerations and any challenges of using different personnel categories as workforce alternatives for meeting operational medical requirements.[108]

To determine the appropriate use of the active and reserve components for DOD's operational medical personnel military requirements, we compared the military departments' efforts in assessing their active and reserve balance to DOD and department-level policies and guidance. Specifically, in a 2013 DOD report issued in response to section 1080A of the National Defense Authorization Act for Fiscal Year 2012, DOD established five factors that play a key role in active and reserve component balance decisions, including the cost of unit manning, training, and equipping. According to the report, cost is often outweighed by other factors when making active component and reserve component mix decisions, but should always be considered in active component and reserve component mix decisions. DOD Instruction 7041.04 has guidance for military departments to use to identify the full cost of their active component, federal civilian, and contractor workforces.[109] Moreover, we interviewed officials from the military departments to discuss: (1) how they determine their operational medical requirements and if they identified the full cost of active and reserve component medical personnel, and (2) the use of the active and reserve components for operational requirements and any efforts to assess the balance of active and reserve component medical personnel.

To determine the mix of active and reserve component medical personnel, we analyzed authorization data from the Health Manpower and Personnel Data System for fiscal year 2017. We analyzed data for fiscal year 2017 because this was the most recent year of available data at the time of our review. To assess the reliability of these data, we electronically tested

---

[108] For this review we selected two combatant commands (U.S. Central Command and U.S. Africa Command) in order to get their perspectives regarding workforce mix in theater.

[109] Department of Defense Instruction 7041.04, *Estimating and Comparing the Full Costs of Civilian and Active Duty Military Manpower and Contract Support* (July 3, 2013).

the data to identify obvious problems with completeness or accuracy and interviewed knowledgeable agency officials about the data. We found the data to be sufficiently reliable for reporting on the allocation of authorizations for active and reserve component medical personnel.

To address how the military departments determine the most appropriate workforce mix at military treatment facilities (MTFs) and any challenges in executing an appropriate workforce mix, we reviewed DOD and department-level policies and guidance on workforce mix determination. We also reviewed the military departments' efforts in planning, staffing, and filling MTF requirements. We spoke with knowledgeable officials from the Office of the USD(P&R), OASD(HA), DHA, and the military departments and requested documentation related to how they oversee or implement legal or policy requirements, such as DOD Instruction 1100.22's manpower mix criteria, and the annual inventory of inherently governmental and commercial activity. To determine the proportion of reported military, federal civilian, and contractor personnel providing or supporting care in MTFs, we obtained budgetary data for fiscal year 2017, which was the most recent full fiscal year of available data at the time of our review. To assess the reliability of these data, we compared them to the information reported in the fiscal year 2017 Defense Health Program justification estimates published in February 2018 to identify key differences and interviewed knowledgeable agency officials about the data. We found the data to be sufficiently reliable for the purposes of describing workforce mix of military, federal civilian, and contractor personnel within MTFs.

To understand how policies and procedures to determine and execute an appropriate workforce mix are implemented at MTFs, we interviewed military department medical command or agency officials responsible for implementing DOD total force policy. To better understand policy and procedure implementation at MTFs we selected six MTFs - two each from the Army, Navy, and Air Force - to allow a cross-section of views concerning the management of the military departments' workforce mix at the MTFs and hiring conditions in different types of labor markets.[110] The two MTFs from each military department were selected based on consideration of average daily patient load and MTF bed size, which we obtained from the Defense Health Agency.

For each MTF, we interviewed officials responsible for the leadership and management of MTF personnel and operations and requested and reviewed relevant documentation. We reviewed their responses, which highlighted some challenges related to achieving an appropriate workforce mix, and DOD's plans for addressing these challenges. We compared these to GAO's key questions to assess agency reform efforts, which note that strategic workforce planning should precede any staff realignments or downsizing,[111] and GAO's key principles for effective strategic workforce planning, which state that addressing a critical human capital challenge—such as closing or reducing personnel gaps—requires tailored human capital strategies and tools and metrics by which to monitor and evaluate progress toward reducing gaps.[112] We also reviewed these plans in light of OPM's standards for strategic workforce planning, which note that human capital strategies should be integrated with acquisition plans, among other things, such as DOD's acquisition strategy for health care services at MTFs.[113] Finally, we requested from officials at each MTF information on personnel inventory and authorizations to understand their ability to fill military and civilian positions, and the contract vendors' ability to fill positions designated for contracted services.

---

[110] We selected the following six MTFs for interviews: (1) Brooke Army Medical Center at Joint Base San Antonio, TX; (2) Carl R. Darnall Army Medical Center in Ft. Hood, TX; (3) Naval Medical Center Portsmouth in Portsmouth, VA; (4) Naval Hospital Twentynine Palms in Twentynine Palms, CA; (5) David Grant Medical Center in Travis AFB, CA; and (6) Air Force Hospital Langley in Hampton, VA.

[111] GAO, *Government Reorganization: Key Questions to Assess Agency Reform Efforts*, GAO-18-427 (Washington, D.C.: June 13, 2018).

[112] GAO-04-39; and 5 C.F.R. § 250.204 (2018).

[113] 5 C.F.R. § 250.203 (2018).

We also reviewed how the planned transfer of administrative responsibility for MTFs from the military departments to the DHA might affect DOD management of military personnel within the MHS. To identify (1) responsibilities of the military departments that may be transferred to the DHA, and (2) challenges that may continue under the new organizational structure, we reviewed relevant documentation and interviewed knowledgeable officials. To understand potential challenges related to the assignment of military personnel to MTFs, we interviewed military department officials responsible for the assignment of military personnel. To identify how deployments affect MTF operations, if at all, we interviewed officials responsible for the leadership and management of MTF personnel and operations. Lastly, to understand how the military departments manage the size and composition of the active duty medical workforce, we requested documentation related to the development of operational personnel requirements and interviewed knowledgeable officials. We also reviewed previous efforts to alter the size or composition of the active duty medical workforce, such as military to civilian conversions. We compared DOD's efforts to plan for these challenges to leading practices for results-oriented government, which state that cooperating federal agencies need to sustain and enhance their collaboration in several ways, including the development of policies and procedures to operate across agency boundaries and agreement on their respective roles and responsibilities.[114]

We conducted this performance audit from September 2017 to November 2018 in accordance with generally accepted government auditing standards. Those standards require that we plan and perform the audit to obtain sufficient, appropriate evidence to provide a reasonable basis for our findings and conclusions based on our audit objectives. We believe that the evidence obtained provides a reasonable basis for our findings and conclusions based on our audit objectives.

---

[114] GAO, *Practices That Can Help Enhance and Sustain Collaboration among Federal Agencies*, GAO-06-15 (Washington, D.C.: Oct. 21, 2005).

Appendix II: Comments from the Department of Defense

OFFICE OF THE ASSISTANT SECRETARY OF DEFENSE
1500 DEFENSE PENTAGON
WASHINGTON, D.C. 20301-4000

MANPOWER AND RESERVE AFFAIRS

NOV - 8 2018

Ms. Brenda Farrell
Director, Defense Capabilities Management
U.S. Government Accountability Office
441 G Street, NW
Washington DC 20548

Dear Ms. Farrell,

This is the Department of Defense (DoD) response to the GAO Draft Report GAO-19-102, "Defense Health Care: Additional Assessments Needed to Better Ensure an Efficient Total Workforce," dated October 5, 2018 (GAO Code 102291).

As you know, the Military Health System (MHS) is the subject of a number of ongoing transformation efforts, as the result not only of internal Departmental reform, but also Congressional oversight and interest. The Department welcomes the GAO's contributions to these efforts, which will help to build a more efficient and effective MHS.

Sincerely,

Lernes Hebert
Acting Director, Total Force Manpower & Resources

GAO DRAFT REPORT DATED OCTOBER 5, 2018
GAO-19-102 (GAO CODE 102291)

"DEFENSE HEALTH CARE: ADDITIONAL ASSESSMENTS NEEDED TO BETTER ENSURE AN EFFICIENT TOTAL WORKFORCE"

DEPARTMENT OF DEFENSE COMMENTS TO THE GAO RECOMMENDATION

RECOMMENDATION 1: The GAO recommends that the Secretary of Defense should ensure that the Assistant Secretary of Defense for Health Affairs, in coordination with the military departments, perform an assessment of the suitability of federal civilian and contractor personnel to provide operation medical care and incorporating the results into relevant policies, if warranted. (Recommendation 1)

DoD RESPONSE: Concur. The Department agrees that assessing the current manpower mix within the Military Health System (MHS) could provide valuable insight into the MHS's overall operations, and identify opportunities for the use of more cost-effective types of labor to accomplish the MHS's missions, as well as the potential for the divestiture of certain services based on cost analysis of network care versus private sector care. This kind of assessment should be iterative, rather than a one-time event, and be an organic part of the requirements determination process used across the MHS, with results being integrated/incorporated, as appropriate, into the Department's programming, planning, budgeting, and execution processes.

RECOMMENDATION 2: The GAO recommends that the Secretary of Defense should ensure that the Under Secretary of Defense for Personnel and Readiness require consideration of cost when making determinations regarding the mix of active and reserve component medical personnel. (Recommendation 2)

DoD RESPONSE: Concur. Cost considerations can be an important factor when determining the most appropriate source of labor to execute a mission or function, and the Department's governing policies for manpower mix and determinations already require consideration not only of cost, but of a variety of factors. As noted in the response to Recommendation 3, below, the Department's governing instruction for costing manpower does not include reserve component military personnel costs, and the inability to include true fully burdened, life-cycle costs of all the types of labor available to the Department inhibits its ability to make informed, cost-effective, and sustainable force mix decisions.

RECOMMENDATION 3: The Secretary of Defense should ensure that the Assistant Secretary of Defense for Health Affairs, in collaboration with the Director of Cost Assessment and Program Evaluation and the military departments, develop full cost information for active and reserve component medical personnel, and the military departments use that information in its determinations regarding the mix of active and reserve component medical personnel. (Recommendation 3)

DoD RESPONSE: Concur. The Department already uses Department of Defense Instruction (DoDI) 7041.04, *Estimating and Comparing the Full Costs of Civilian and Active Duty Military Manpower and Contractor Support* for determining the cost of active component military personnel, though it does not address determination of cost for reserve component military personnel.

RECOMMENDATION 4: The GAO recommends that the Secretary of Defense should ensure that the Director of the DHA develop a strategic total workforce plan which includes, among other things: (1) tailored human capital strategies, tools, and metrics by which to monitor and evaluate progress toward reducing personnel gaps, and; (2) integration of human capital strategies with acquisition plans, such as DOD's acquisition strategy for health care services at DOD's military treatment facilities. (Recommendation 4)

DoD RESPONSE: Concur. The Department agrees that the recommended considerations are critical to strategic total workforce planning, and that any plan needs to take into account the unique particulars surrounding the MHS, so as to avoid a "one-size-fits-all" solution. Additionally, strategic total workforce planning should be part of an iterative process, integrated with and complementary to the Department's programming, planning, budgeting, and execution processes rather than a one-time event or stand-alone product.

RECOMMENDATION 5: The GAO recommends that the Secretary of Defense and the Secretaries of the Army, the Navy, and the Air Force, respectively, should ensure that accompanying the transfer of MTFs to the DHA, that the DHA and the military departments develop policies and procedure for management of military personnel, including agreement on specific roles and responsibilities for the departments and the DHA in this process. (Recommendation 5)

DoD RESPONSE: Concur. The Department agrees that policies and procedures for managing military personnel throughout the transition of MTFs are necessary, though this issue can be handled within existing business processes and does not necessarily need to be elevated to the level of the Service Secretaries or Secretary of Defense.

In: Defense Health Care
Editor: Frederick Duncan

ISBN: 978-1-53615-175-6

Chapter 4

DEFENSE HEALTH CARE: TRICARE SURVEYS INDICATE NONENROLLED BENEFICIARIES' ACCESS TO CARE HAS GENERALLY IMPROVED*

United States Government Accountability Office

ABBREVIATIONS

CAHPS	Consumer Assessment of Healthcare Providers and Systems
DOD	Department of Defense
HHS	Department of Health and Human Services
HSA	Hospital Service Area
NDAA	National Defense Authorization Act
NDAA 2008	National Defense Authorization Act for

* This is an edited, reformatted and augmented version of United States Government Accountability Office; Report to Congressional Committees, Publication No. GAO-18-361, dated March 2018.

	Fiscal Year 2008
NDAA 2012	National Defense Authorization Act for Fiscal Year 2012
NDAA 2017	National Defense Authorization Act for Fiscal Year 2017
PSA	Prime Service Area
VA	Department of Veterans Affairs

WHY GAO DID THIS STUDY

DOD provides health care, including mental health care, to eligible beneficiaries through TRICARE. Beneficiaries who use TRICARE Prime, a managed care option, must enroll to receive care. Prior to Jan. 1, 2018, beneficiaries did not need to enroll for TRICARE Standard, a fee- for-service option, or TRICARE Extra, a preferred provider organization option (referred to as nonenrolled beneficiaries). Although the TRICARE Standard and Extra options were terminated effective Jan. 1, 2018, the new TRICARE Select option has similar benefits for obtaining care from network and nonnetwork providers.

The National Defense Authorization Act (NDAA) for Fiscal Year 2008 directed DOD to conduct surveys of nonenrolled beneficiaries and civilian providers about access to care under the TRICARE Standard and Extra options. It also directed GAO to review the surveys' results. Additionally, the NDAA for Fiscal Year 2017 included a provision for GAO to review access to care under TRICARE Extra. This chapter addresses both provisions.

GAO analyzed DOD's surveys to determine (1) nonenrolled beneficiaries' access to care, (2) nonenrolled beneficiaries' ratings of TRICARE, (3) civilian providers' awareness and acceptance of TRICARE, and (4) nonenrolled beneficiaries' access by individual geographic area. GAO interviewed agency officials, analyzed the 2012-2015 surveys, and compared them to DOD's 2008-2011 surveys and to surveys of Medicare and Medicaid beneficiaries. In commenting on a draft of this chapter, DOD concurred with GAO's findings.

What GAO Found

The Department of Defense's (DOD) most recent surveys of TRICARE beneficiaries and civilian health care providers show that access to care has generally improved for nonenrolled beneficiaries who used the TRICARE Standard and Extra options. Specifically, GAO found the following:

- Nonenrolled beneficiaries reported improved access to care in the most recent 4-year survey (2012-2015), compared to the prior survey (2008-2011). For example, a lower percentage of nonenrolled beneficiaries reported that they experienced problems finding a civilian provider in the most recent survey (29 percent) than those in the prior survey (31 percent). In addition, a higher percentage of nonenrolled beneficiaries (90 percent) reported that they were usually or always able to obtain a non-urgent appointment as soon as they thought they needed compared to the prior survey (87 percent).
- The percentage of nonenrolled beneficiaries who reported positive experience ratings of TRICARE ranged from 71 to 83 percent over five categories, including ratings of primary, specialty, and mental health care providers. These ratings were generally higher than the prior survey. When compared to other federal health plans, nonenrolled TRICARE beneficiaries' positive experience ratings of primary and specialty care providers were lower than those of Medicare fee-for service beneficiaries, but higher than those of Medicaid beneficiaries.
- The percentage of civilian providers who were aware of TRICARE increased from 82 percent in the prior survey to 84 percent. However, the percentage who accepted new TRICARE patients decreased from 58 percent to 55 percent. According to GAO's

analysis of survey data, this overall decrease was mainly attributable to a decrease in mental health care providers' acceptance rates, as the acceptance rates for primary and specialty care providers remained unchanged. Network providers reported both higher awareness and acceptance of TRICARE than providers not in the network (referred to as nonnetwork providers). The biggest gap in both awareness and acceptance between network and nonnetwork providers was for mental health care providers:

- o About 96 percent of network mental health care providers reported awareness of TRICARE compared to 72 percent of nonnetwork mental health care providers.
- o About 79 percent of network mental health care providers reported accepting new TRICARE patients compared to 30 percent of nonnetwork mental health care providers.

- GAO's analysis of both the beneficiary and provider surveys identified locations in New York, Washington, Texas, and Washington, D.C. where access to providers may be particularly problematic. Specifically, in these locations, beneficiaries reported more problems finding providers who accepted TRICARE and providers reported lower acceptance of TRICARE, compared to national averages.

March 29, 2018

The Honorable John McCain
Chairman

The Honorable Jack Reed
Ranking Minority Member
Committee on Armed Services
United States Senate

The Honorable Mac Thornberry
Chairman

The Honorable Adam Smith
Ranking Minority Member
Committee on Armed Services
House of Representatives

In fiscal year 2016, the Department of Defense (DOD) offered health care services, including mental health care, to more than 9 million eligible beneficiaries in the United States and abroad through TRICARE, DOD's regionally structured health care program.[1] Under TRICARE, beneficiaries may obtain care either from military hospitals and clinics, referred to collectively as military treatment facilities, or from civilian providers.[2] However, since TRICARE's inception in 1995, beneficiaries in some locations—particularly those who did not enroll in TRICARE's managed care option—have raised concerns about difficulties finding civilian providers who will accept them as patients.

The number and type of civilian providers available to serve TRICARE beneficiaries can vary depending on a beneficiary's location and choice of coverage—which prior to January 1, 2018, consisted of TRICARE's three basic plans: Prime, Extra, and Standard.[3] Beneficiaries who used TRICARE Prime, a managed care option, had to enroll and could obtain care through military treatment facilities or TRICARE's network of civilian providers.[4] DOD uses contractors, called managed care support contractors, to develop networks of civilian providers (network providers) to ensure adequate access to care for all TRICARE beneficiaries in geographic areas called Prime Service Areas (PSA).[5] Although some network providers may be located

---

[1] Eligible beneficiaries include active duty personnel and their dependents, medically eligible National Guard and Reserve servicemembers and their dependents, and retirees and their dependents and survivors, among others. Active duty personnel include Reserve component members on active duty for at least 30 days.

[2] Through individual agreements between military treatment facilities and the Department of Veterans Affairs' (VA) medical centers, eligible beneficiaries also may receive certain types of care from VA medical centers in some locations.

[3] The National Defense Authorization Act for Fiscal Year 2017 included a number of changes to the TRICARE program, including the termination of TRICARE Standard and Extra and the establishment of a new option, TRICARE Select, which took effect on Jan. 1, 2018.

[4] Active duty personnel are required to use TRICARE Prime.

[5] PSAs are defined by a set of five-digit zip codes, usually within an approximate 40-mile radius of a military outpatient or inpatient treatment facility or a Base Realignment and Closure site,

outside of PSAs, contractors are not required to develop networks in these areas (which we refer to as non- PSAs).

Beneficiaries did not need to enroll to receive care under TRICARE Standard, a fee-for-service option, or TRICARE Extra, a preferred provider organization option. These beneficiaries—referred to as nonenrolled beneficiaries—could choose to receive care either through TRICARE Standard when they saw nonnetwork civilian providers or through TRICARE Extra when they saw network civilian providers. The National Defense Authorization Act for Fiscal Year 2017 (NDAA 2017) terminated both the TRICARE Standard and Extra options and established a self-managed preferred provider option called TRICARE Select beginning January 1, 2018.

In response to nonenrolled beneficiaries' concerns about access to care, the National Defense Authorization Act for Fiscal Year 2008 (NDAA 2008) directed DOD to conduct a multi-year survey (2008-2011) of nonenrolled beneficiaries and a multi-year survey (2008-2011) of civilian providers to determine the adequacy of access to health care providers, including mental health care providers, for nonenrolled beneficiaries.[6] The National Defense Authorization Act for Fiscal Year 2012 (NDAA 2012) directed DOD to continue both of these surveys for an additional 4-year period (2012-2015).[7]

The NDAA 2008 also included a recurring provision for us to review a series of issues related to the adequacy of access to care for nonenrolled TRICARE beneficiaries, including information gleaned from the beneficiary and civilian provider surveys, and to report on these issues on a biannual basis.[8] We have issued a series of reports in response to this provision, including two reports that focused on DOD's beneficiary and civilian provider surveys.[9] In addition, the NDAA 2017 directed us to conduct a

---

which is a military installation that has been closed or realigned as a result of decisions made by the Commission on Base Realignment and Closure.

[6] See Pub. L. No. 110-181, § 711(a), 122 Stat. 3, 190-191. (2008).

[7] Pub. L. No. 112-81, § 721(a), 125 Stat. 1298, 1478 (2011).

[8] This reporting time frame was amended in the NDAA 2012 to biennial reporting instead of biannual reporting. The National Defense Authorization Act for Fiscal Year 2015 amended GAO's reporting requirements to issue two remaining reports—one in 2017 and one in 2020.

[9] For the reports on DOD's surveys, see GAO, *Defense Health Care: TRICARE Multiyear Surveys Indicate Problems with Access to Care for Nonenrolled Beneficiaries*, GAO-13-364

review of the network of civilian providers that provide care to nonenrolled beneficiaries under the TRICARE Extra option.[10]

This chapter addresses provisions in both the NDAA 2008, as amended, and the NDAA 2017 for us to report on the adequacy of access to care for nonenrolled TRICARE beneficiaries. Specifically, it describes

1) what the results of the most recent 4-year beneficiary survey indicate about access to care for nonenrolled beneficiaries;
2) what the results of the most recent 4-year beneficiary survey indicate about nonenrolled beneficiaries' ratings of their experience with TRICARE;
3) what the results of the most recent 4-year civilian provider survey indicate about civilian providers' awareness and acceptance of TRICARE; and
4) what the collective results of the most recent 4-year beneficiary and civilian provider surveys indicate about access to care for nonenrolled beneficiaries by geographic area.

To determine what the results of the most recent 4-year beneficiary survey indicate about access to care for nonenrolled beneficiaries, we obtained and analyzed survey data from DOD's TRICARE Standard Surveys of Beneficiaries for 2012-2015. Specifically, we analyzed these data to determine whether nonenrolled beneficiaries were able to obtain an appointment as soon as they wanted, how quickly they were able to get an appointment to see a provider, and if they had a problem finding a provider

(Washington, D.C.: Apr. 2, 2013) and *Defense Health Care: 2008 Access to Care Surveys Indicate Some Problems, but Beneficiary Satisfaction Is Similar to Other Health Plans*, GAO-10-402 (Washington, D.C.: Mar. 31, 2010). Other reports in response to this provision include *Defense Health Care: More-Specific Guidance Needed for Assessing Nonenrolled TRICARE Beneficiaries' Access to Care*, GAO-14-384 (Washington, D.C.: Apr. 28, 2014); *Defense Health Care: DOD Lacks Assurance That Selected Reserve Members Are Informed About TRICARE Reserve Select*, GAO-11-551 (Washington, D.C.: June 3, 2011); and *Defense Health Care: Access to Civilian Providers under TRICARE Standard and Extra*, GAO-11-500 (Washington, D.C.: June 2, 2011).

[10] Pub. L. No. 114-328, § 701(g)(2), 130 Stat. 2000, 2188 (2016).

that would accept TRICARE.[11] We compared these data across location types, provider types, and providers' network status, where applicable. We also compared these results to DOD's 2008-2011 survey results to identify any changes in beneficiaries' access over time.

To determine what the results of the most recent 4-year beneficiary survey indicate about nonenrolled beneficiaries' ratings of their experience with TRICARE, we obtained and analyzed the 2012-2015 nonenrolled beneficiary survey data that indicated beneficiaries' ratings of certain aspects of their TRICARE experiences, such as their ratings of health care, health plan, and primary, specialty, and mental health care providers.[12] We compared these data by providers' network status, where applicable. We also obtained and analyzed data from the Department of Health and Human Services' (HHS) Consumer Assessment of Healthcare Providers and Systems (CAHPS) surveys for the 2013-2015 time period to compare nonenrolled TRICARE beneficiaries' ratings to those of Medicare fee-for-service and Medicaid beneficiaries.[13] Additionally, we compared the results of DOD's 2012-2015 beneficiary surveys to DOD's 2008-2011 survey results to identify any changes in beneficiaries' ratings of experiences over time. To determine what the results of the most recent 4-year civilian provider surveys indicate about civilian providers' awareness and acceptance of TRICARE, we obtained and analyzed survey data from DOD's TRICARE Standard Surveys of Providers for 2012-2015. We compared these data by location type, provider type, and providers' network status, where applicable. We compared these results to the results from

[11] For mental health care, the survey question asked beneficiaries how much of a problem it was to get the "treatment or counseling you needed through your health plan," and not necessarily to find a provider that would accept TRICARE.

[12] DOD reports beneficiaries' ratings as positive if they are on an 8, 9, or 10 on a 0-10 point scale. We did the same in our analysis.

[13] DOD based its nonenrolled beneficiary survey questions on HHS's CAHPS survey, which allows for comparisons between the surveys. HHS's CAHPS survey is an annual, national survey of beneficiaries of commercial health insurance, Medicare, Medicaid, and the Children's Health Insurance Program. According to a CAHPS official, the CAHPS survey for Medicare and Medicaid beneficiaries was not conducted in 2012. Therefore, for each of the Medicare fee-for-service and Medicaid surveys, we combined the 2013-2015 annual data into one point estimate in order to compare the results to DOD's 4-year beneficiary surveys over a similar period.

DOD's 2008-2011 surveys to identify any changes in provider awareness and acceptance over time.

To determine what the collective results of the most recent 4-year beneficiary and civilian provider surveys indicate about access to care for nonenrolled beneficiaries, we compared the results of our analyses of the 2012-2015 beneficiary and provider survey data by specific geographic regions, where possible, in order to identify locations with high percentages of nonenrolled beneficiaries who experienced problems finding civilian providers and low percentages of civilian providers who were accepting new TRICARE patients.[14] We conducted this analysis by individual location type and provider type.

For each objective, we assessed the reliability of the data from the surveys–including DOD's 2012-2015 nonenrolled beneficiary and civilian provider surveys and HHS's CAHPS survey–by speaking with knowledgeable officials and reviewing relevant documentation. DOD calculated the response rates for its 2012-2015 nonenrolled beneficiary surveys and civilian provider surveys to be about 25 percent and 39 percent, respectively.[15] We verified that the surveys' results were representative of the areas surveyed by reviewing DOD's nonresponse analyses for these surveys and by interviewing DOD officials.[16] We determined that all data

---

[14] Similar to our report on the prior 4-year surveys, we correlated survey results for which both (1) beneficiaries reported more problems finding civilian providers than the national average and (2) civilian providers reported less acceptance of new TRICARE patients than the national average. See GAO-13-364.

[15] For the 4 years of the nonenrolled beneficiary survey, DOD mailed 146,125 surveys and received 35,242 complete and eligible responses, 19,415 of which were from nonenrolled TRICARE beneficiaries. DOD considered complete and eligible responses as those where TRICARE beneficiaries who answered at least half of the DOD-identified "key" questions. Over the 4 years of the 2012-2015 civilian provider survey, DOD mailed 192,129 surveys to physician and mental health providers, and received 50,331 complete and eligible responses. DOD considered the survey complete if the provider answered three DOD- identified "key" questions that asked about the providers' locations of practice and awareness and acceptance of TRICARE.

[16] DOD concluded that the results of thc beneficiary survey nonresponse analyses suggested that although there were some differences in the demographic profiles between respondents and nonrespondents, they were not associated with systematic differences in satisfaction with care.

From the results of the civilian provider survey nonresponse analyses, DOD concluded that there were only slight differences between respondents and nonrespondents in terms of the type of provider. For both the beneficiary and provider surveys, DOD officials also told us

used in this chapter were sufficiently reliable for our purposes. However, our analyses have some limitations. In our collective analyses of DOD's beneficiary and provider surveys, we were not able to compare survey results among all of the individual geographic locations due to low numbers of respondents in some areas. Specifically, we excluded individual locations that had less than 30 respondents to the beneficiary survey or less than 50 respondents to the provider survey, depending on the survey questions we analyzed. Due to the low numbers of respondents who indicated that they needed mental health care, we were unable to identify specific geographic locations in which nonenrolled beneficiaries experienced problems finding mental health providers.

We conducted this performance audit from March 2017 to March 2018 in accordance with generally accepted government auditing standards. Those standards require that we plan and perform the audit to obtain sufficient, appropriate evidence to provide a reasonable basis for our findings and conclusions based on our audit objectives. We believe that the evidence obtained provides a reasonable basis for our findings and conclusions based on our audit objectives.

BACKGROUND

Composition of TRICARE's Nonenrolled Beneficiary Population

In fiscal year 2016, DOD identified about 2.2 million nonenrolled TRICARE beneficiaries who fell into four categories: (1) retired servicemembers and their dependents, (2) inactive guard/reserve servicemembers and their dependents, (3) dependents of active duty, or of guard/reserve on active duty status, and (4) other beneficiaries, such as dependent survivors of deceased servicemembers. Retired servicemembers

---

that the final post-survey weights used in their analyses accounted for the key characteristic differences in survey respondents compared with nonrespondents identified through the nonresponse analyses for both types of surveys.

and their dependents made up the majority of nonenrolled beneficiaries at the end of fiscal year 2016 (approximately 60 percent) (See Figure 1).

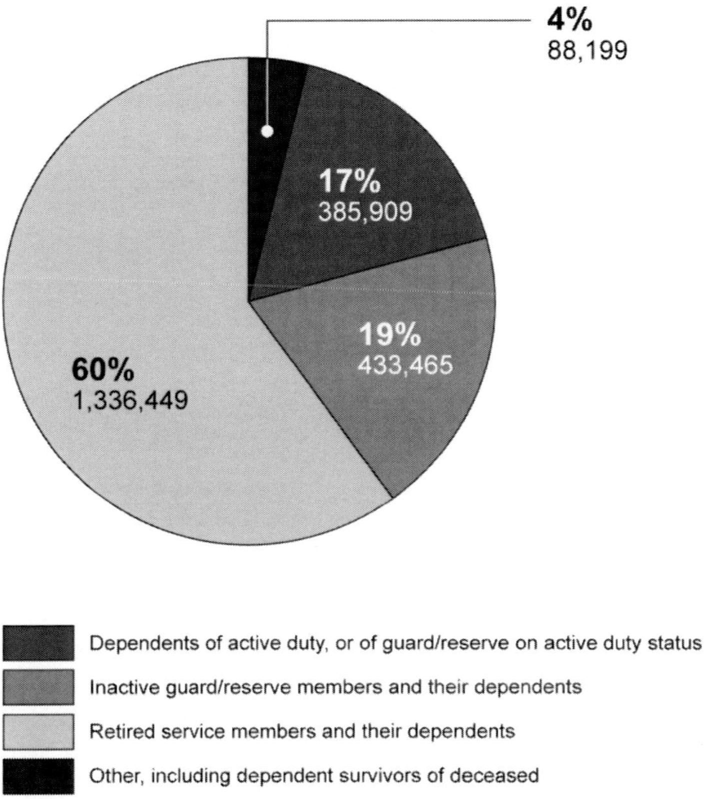

Source: GAO analysis of Department of Defense data. | GAO-18-361.

Figure 1. Percentage of Nonenrolled TRICARE Beneficiaries by Beneficiary Category, September 2016 (Number of Beneficiaries).

TRICARE's Benefit Options

Prior to January 1, 2018, TRICARE provided benefits through three basic options for its non-Medicare-eligible beneficiary population—

TRICARE Prime, Standard, and Extra.[17] These options varied by enrollment requirements, choices in civilian and military treatment facility providers, and the amount beneficiaries must contribute toward the cost of their care (See Table 1).

Table 1. Summary of Basic TRICARE Options Prior to January 1, 2018

TRICARE option	Description
TRICARE Prime	This is TRICARE's managed care option and requires enrollment. All active duty servicemembers are required to use this option, while other TRICARE beneficiaries may choose it. Prime enrollees receive most of their care from providers at military treatment facilities and also may receive care from network civilian providers. This option has the lowest out-of-pocket costs for beneficiaries, as care provided at military treatment facilities does not have an associated copayment.
TRICARE Standard and Extra	TRICARE beneficiaries who chose not to enroll in TRICARE Prime were able to obtain health care from nonnetwork providers (TRICARE Standard) or network civilian providers (TRICARE Extra). The TRICARE Standard option was designed to provide beneficiaries with maximum flexibility in selecting providers, but beneficiaries who obtained care from a network provider through TRICARE Extra paid lower copayments than they would if they had chosen a nonnetwork provider under the TRICARE Standard option. TRICARE Standard and Extra beneficiaries could also receive care from military treatment facilities, though they had a lower priority for receiving care than TRICARE Prime beneficiaries.

Source: GAO summary of Department of Defense TRICARE documentation. | GAO-18-361.

The NDAA 2017 made specific changes to the TRICARE program that became effective on January 1, 2018. These changes included terminating the TRICARE Standard and Extra options, establishing a new option called

[17] TRICARE also offers TRICARE for Life to TRICARE beneficiaries who are eligible for Medicare and enroll in Part B. Under the TRICARE for Life program, TRICARE processes claims after they have been adjudicated by Medicare.

TRICARE Select, and ensuring that 85 percent of TRICARE Select beneficiaries are covered by the network of civilian providers.

TRICARE Select has similar benefits to TRICARE Standard and Extra for obtaining care from nonnetwork and network providers, but unlike these options, TRICARE Select requires enrollment.

TRICARE Networks and Locations

Under TRICARE, DOD uses managed care support contractors to develop networks of civilian providers to serve all TRICARE beneficiaries in PSAs, which are typically within an approximate 40-mile radius of a military outpatient or inpatient treatment facility or Base Realignment and Closure sites. Although some network providers may be located in non-PSAs, contractors are not required to develop networks in these areas. Previously, contractors had the option of developing additional PSAs (and civilian provider networks) in areas that were not located near military treatment facilities or Base Realignment and Closure sites. However, on October 1, 2013, DOD eliminated these additional PSAs, referred to in the survey analyses as "former PSAs," and as a result, the managed care support contractors were no longer required to develop and maintain networks of civilian providers in these areas.[18]

In fiscal year 2016, approximately 65 percent of the 2.2 million nonenrolled beneficiaries that were eligible for TRICARE Standard and Extra (1.47 million) lived in PSAs. Of the remaining nonenrolled beneficiaries (775,000), about 19 percent lived in former PSAs and about 16 percent lived in non-PSAs (See Figure 2). Nonenrolled beneficiaries who live in former PSAs and non-PSAs may still have access to network providers, even though contractors are not required to develop networks in these areas. About 57 percent of these beneficiaries (445,000) filed at least one TRICARE claim with a network civilian provider during fiscal year 2016.

---

[18] Managed care support contractor officials told us that they did not have plans to eliminate the networks of providers that were already established in those locations.

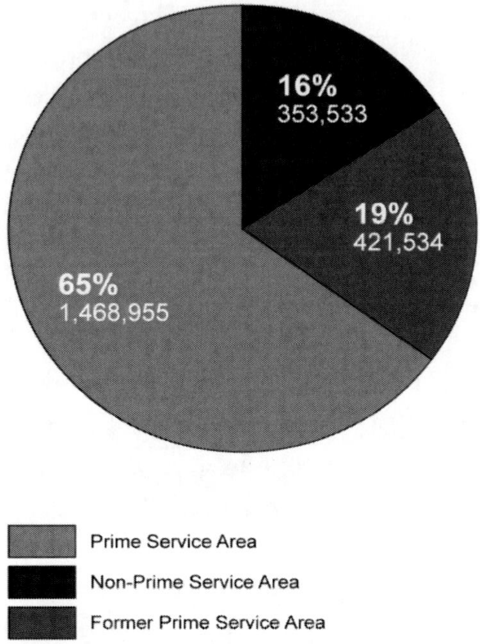

Source: GAO analysis of Department of Defense data. | GAO-18-361.

Note: The Department of Defense requires its TRICARE contractors to develop networks of civilian providers (network providers) in geographic areas called Prime Service Areas, which are defined by a set of five-digit zip codes, usually within an approximate 40-mile radius of a military outpatient or inpatient treatment facility or a Base Realignment and Closure site. Contractors are not required to develop networks outside of these areas, which we refer to as non-Prime Service Areas. Previously, contractors had the option of developing additional Prime Service Areas (and civilian provider networks), in areas that were not located near military treatment facilities or Base Realignment and Closure sites. However, on Oct. 1, 2013, DOD eliminated these additional areas, which are referred to as "former Prime Service Areas."

Figure 2. Percentage of Nonenrolled TRICARE Beneficiaries by Location, September 2016 (Number of Beneficiaries).

DOD's Implementation of Mandated Beneficiary and Civilian Provider Survey Requirements

The NDAA 2008 directed DOD to survey nonenrolled beneficiaries and civilian providers in at least 20 PSAs in each of four fiscal years, 2008 through 2011, as well as 20 non-PSAs. To do this, DOD divided the country into 80 distinct PSAs and 80 distinct non-PSAs and surveyed 20 PSAs and 20 non-PSAs each year. At the end of the 4-year period, each year's survey results were combined and weighted to develop estimates of access to health care, including mental health care, at the service area, state, and national levels. Additionally, the NDAA 2008 required DOD to consult with representatives of TRICARE beneficiaries and providers of health care, including mental health care, to identify locations where nonenrolled beneficiaries have experienced significant access-to-care problems and to survey both beneficiaries and health care providers, including mental health care providers, in these areas. Based on these consultations, DOD designated certain Hospital Service Areas (HSA) to include in its beneficiary and provider surveys.[19]

DOD used a similar methodology for determining its locations in the 2012-2015 surveys. However, as a result of DOD's changes to PSAs on October 1, 2013, 28 of the 80 non-PSAs surveyed were former PSAs. DOD also surveyed both nonenrolled beneficiaries and civilian providers in a total of 30 HSAs. As a result, DOD collectively surveyed 190 geographic locations over the 4-year period.[20] Furthermore, we previously reported that DOD's implementation of its 2008-2011 nonenrolled beneficiary and civilian provider surveys generally addressed the requirements outlined in the NDAA 2008.[21] DOD made several minor revisions to the methodologies of the 2012-2015 surveys, but we determined that none of those changes altered DOD's compliance with the NDAA 2008, as amended.

---

[19] According to DOD officials, representatives of TRICARE beneficiaries and health care providers suggested cities and towns where access should be measured, and DOD then identified HSAs corresponding to each city and town. HSAs, as defined by a Dartmouth University study, are collections of zip codes organized into more than 3,000 geographic regions in which Medicare beneficiaries seek the majority of their care from one hospital or a collection of hospitals. HSAs have non-overlapping borders and contain all U.S. zip codes without gaps in coverage. The HSAs included in the beneficiary and civilian provider surveys are within the PSAs or non-PSAs surveyed.

[20] The 80 PSAs, 52 non-PSAs, and 28 former PSAs covered the entire country. Even though the 30 HSAs are contained within the surveyed PSAs, non-PSAs, or former PSAs, DOD counts them as separate locations, totaling 190 surveyed areas.

[21] See GAO-10-402 and GAO-13-364. For more detailed information on DOD's methodology for the surveys, see Appendix II in GAO-10-402 and Appendix I in GAO-13-364.

NONENROLLED TRICARE BENEFICIARIES REPORTED GENERALLY EXPERIENCING FEWER PROBLEMS ACCESSING CARE, AND MORE REPORTED OBTAINING CARE WHEN DESIRED

Nonenrolled TRICARE Beneficiaries Reported Generally Experiencing Fewer Problems Accessing Care Than in the Prior Survey

Nonenrolled Beneficiary Survey Results over Time

Nonenrolled TRICARE beneficiaries who reported they experienced problems accessing a TRICARE provider were surveyed on the reasons for their problems. "Dr. was not accepting TRICARE payment" was the most-reported reason among all three provider types—primary care, specialty care, and mental health—and was reported by about 50 percent of respondents.

Some of the other top reasons reported were that the

- doctor was not taking any new TRICARE
- patients;
- doctor was not taking any new patients;
- travel distance was too long; or
- wait time for an appointment was too long

These top reasons were similar for both network and nonnetwork providers.

Source: GAO analysis of Department of Defense data. | GAO-18-361.

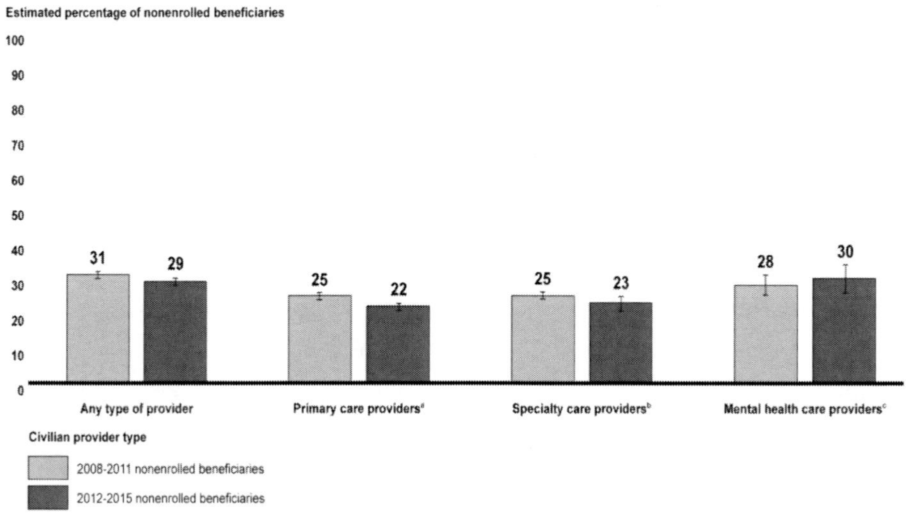

Source: GAO analysis of Department of Defense data. | GAO-18-361.

Notes: Bars display 95 percent confidence levels for estimates, rounded to a whole number. Within provider types, the differences in estimates between the 2008-2011 survey and the 2012-2015 survey are statistically different at the 95 percent confidence level for "any type of provider" and primary care providers.

[a]Respondents answered "a big problem" or "a small problem" to the question that asked: In the last 12 months, how much of a problem was it to find a personal doctor who would accept TRICARE? Answer choices were "a big problem," "a small problem," or "not a problem."

[b]Respondents answered "a big problem" or "a small problem" to the question that asked: "In the last 12 months, how much of a problem was it to find a doctor with this specialty who would accept TRICARE? Answer choices were "a big problem," "a small problem," or "not a problem."

[c]Respondents answered "a big problem" or "a small problem" to the question that asked: "In the last 12 months, how much of a problem, if any, was it to get the treatment or counseling you needed through your health plan? Answer choices were "a big problem," "a small problem," or "not a problem."

Figure 3. Nonenrolled TRICARE Beneficiaries Who Reported Experiencing Problems Finding a Civilian Provider over Time, by Provider Type.

Specifically, fewer nonenrolled beneficiaries reported that they experienced problems finding a primary care provider than in the prior survey (22 percent in 2012-2015 compared to 25 percent in 2008-2011).[22]

However, there was no significant statistical difference over time in the percentage of beneficiaries who reported experiencing problems finding a specialty care or mental health care provider (See Figure 3).

Nonenrolled Beneficiary Survey Results by Type of Location

Nonenrolled beneficiaries in non-PSAs reported experiencing fewer problems finding primary and specialty providers than those in PSAs, which is similar to what we reported for the prior survey.[23] For example, about 20 percent of beneficiaries in non-PSAs reported that they had problems finding specialty care providers compared to 24 percent in PSAs.[24] Regarding beneficiaries in former PSAs, the only statistically significant difference among the three provider types was for problems finding a primary care provider. Specifically, fewer (about 19 percent) nonenrolled beneficiaries in non-PSAs reported experiencing problems finding a primary care provider to accept TRICARE, compared to 24 percent in former PSAs[25] (See Figure 4). DOD officials told us that they were unsure of the exact reasons for the difference between PSAs and non- PSAs. However, they explained that PSAs are often located in more populated areas, where TRICARE beneficiaries may not make up a large market share for local civilian providers, who may have a wide array of patients with other health plans.

---

[22] The margins of error for the estimates of beneficiary problems finding civilian primary care providers are within plus or minus 1 percentage point at the 95 percent confidence level. The difference in estimates is significant at the 95 percent confidence level.

[23] See GAO-13-364.

[24] The margins of error for these estimates are within plus or minus 2 percentage points at the 95 percent confidence level. The difference in estimates is significant at the 95 percent confidence level.

[25] The margins of error for these estimates are within plus or minus 3 percentage points at the 95 percent confidence level. The difference in estimates is significant at the 95 percent confidence level.

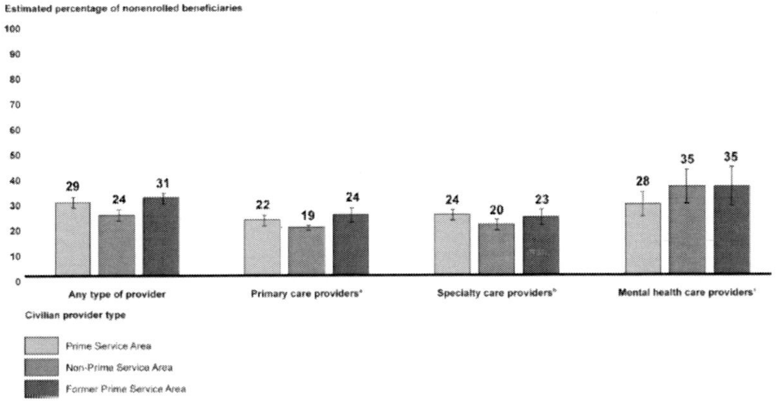

Source: GAO analysis of Department of Defense data. | GAO-18-361.

Notes: Bars display 95 percent confidence levels for estimates, rounded to a whole number. The Department of Defense requires its TRICARE contractors to develop networks of civilian providers (network providers) in geographic areas called Prime Service Areas, which are defined by a set of five-digit zip codes, usually within an approximate 40-mile radius of a military outpatient or inpatient treatment facility or a Base Realignment and Closure site. Contractors are not required to develop networks outside of these areas, which we refer to as non-Prime Service Areas. Previously, contractors had the option of developing additional Prime Service Areas (and civilian provider networks), in areas that were not located near military treatment facilities or Base Realignment and Closure sites. However, on October 1, 2013, DOD eliminated these additional areas, which are referred to as "former Prime Service Areas." Within provider types, the following differences in estimates between location types are statistically different at the 95 percent confidence level: within "any type of provider" and primary care providers, the estimates for non-Prime Service Areas are less than those for Prime Service Areas or former Prime Service Areas; within specialty care providers, the estimate for non-Prime Service Areas is less than Prime Service Areas.

[a]Respondents answered "a big problem" or "a small problem" to the question that asked: In the last 12 months, how much of a problem was it to find a personal doctor who would accept TRICARE? Answer choices were "a big problem," "a small problem," or "not a problem."

[b]Respondents answered "a big problem" or "a small problem" to the question that asked: "In the last 12 months, how much of a problem was it to find a doctor with this specialty who would accept TRICARE? Answer choices were "a big problem," "a small problem," or "not a problem."

[c]Respondents answered "a big problem" or "a small problem" to the question that asked: Based on the following: In the last 12 months, how much of a problem, if any, was it to get the treatment or counseling you needed through your health plan? Answer choices were "a big problem," "a small problem," or "not a problem."

Figure 4. Nonenrolled TRICARE Beneficiaries Who Reported Experiencing Problems Finding a Civilian Provider, by Provider Type and Location Type (2012-2015).

Nonenrolled Beneficiary Survey Results by Network Status

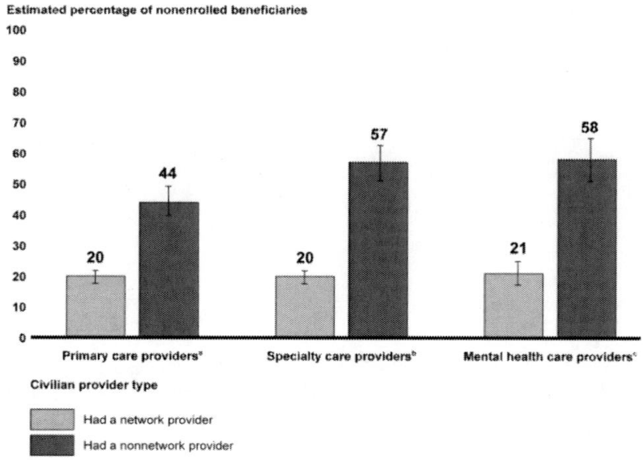

Source: GAO analysis of Department of Defense data. | GAO-18-361.

Notes: Bars display 95 percent confidence levels for estimates, rounded to a whole number.

Within each provider type, the differences in estimates between network and nonnetwork providers are statistically different at the 95 percent confidence level.

Due to the wording of the questions, we could not determine the problems finding "any type of provider" by network status.

[a]For the providers' network status, respondents answered either "yes" or "no" to the question that asked: Is your personal doctor part of the TRICARE civilian provider network? In addition, respondents answered either "a big problem" or "a small problem" to the question that asked: In the last 12 months, how much of a problem was it to find a personal doctor who would accept TRICARE? Answer choices were "a big problem," "a small problem," or "not a problem."

[b]For the providers' network status, respondents answered either "yes" or "no" to the question that asked: In the last 12 months, was the civilian specialist you saw most part of the TRICARE civilian provider network? In addition, respondents answered "a big problem" or "a small problem" to the question that asked: "In the last 12 months, how much of a problem was it to find a doctor with this specialty who would accept TRICARE? Answer choices were "a big problem," "a small problem," or "not a problem."

[c]For the providers' network status, respondents answered either "yes" or "no" to the question that asked: In the last 12 months, did you receive this treatment or counseling from a provider in TRICARE's civilian network? In addition, respondents answered "a big problem" or "a small problem" to the question that asked: Based on the following: In the last 12 months, how much of a problem, if any, was it to get the treatment or counseling you needed through your health plan? Answer choices were "a big problem," "a small problem," or "not a problem."

Figure 5. Nonenrolled TRICARE Beneficiaries Who Reported Experiencing Problems Finding a Civilian Provider, by Provider Type and Network Status (2012-2015).

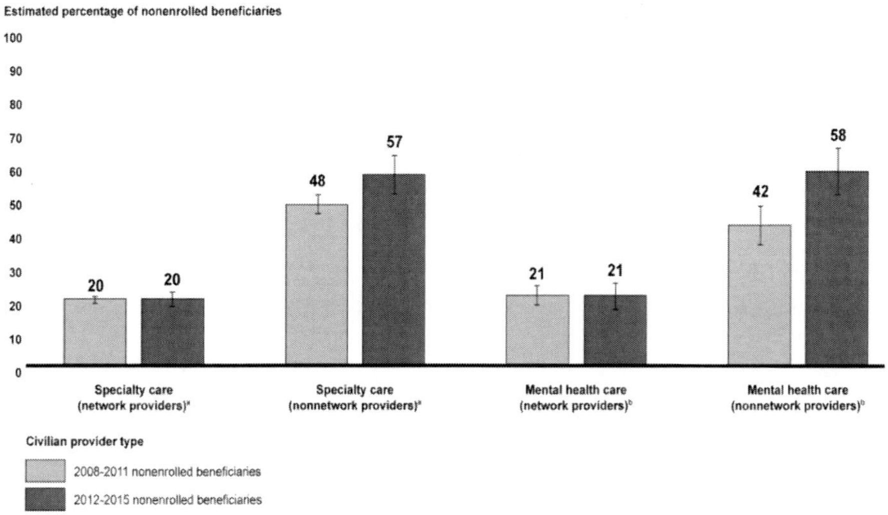

Source: GAO analysis of Department of Defense data. | GAO-18-361.

Notes: Bars display 95 percent confidence levels for estimates, rounded to a whole number. Within specialty health care and mental health care nonnetwork providers, the differences in estimates between the 2008-2011 and 2012-2015 surveys are statistically different at the 95 percent confidence level.

[a]For the providers' network status, respondents answered either "yes" or "no" to the question that asked: In the last 12 months, was the civilian specialist you saw most part of the TRICARE civilian provider network? In addition, respondents answered "a big problem" or "a small problem" to the question that asked: In the last 12 months, how much of a problem was it to find a doctor with this specialty who would accept TRICARE? Answer choices were "a big problem," "a small problem," or "not a problem."

[b]For the providers' network status, respondents answered either "yes" or "no" to the question that asked: In the last 12 months, did you receive this treatment or counseling from a provider in TRICARE's civilian network? In addition, respondents answered "a big problem" or "a small problem" to the question that asked: Based on the following: In the last 12 months, how much of a problem, if any, was it to get the treatment or counseling you needed through your health plan? Answer choices were "a big problem," "a small problem," or "not a problem."

Figure 6. Nonenrolled TRICARE Beneficiaries Who Reported Experiencing Problems Finding a Specialty or Mental Health Care Provider over Time, by Provider Type and Network Status.

Nonenrolled beneficiaries with network providers reported experiencing fewer problems finding civilian providers, compared to nonenrolled beneficiaries with nonnetwork providers. For example, 20 percent of the nonenrolled beneficiaries who used a network civilian primary care provider reported that they had a problem finding a primary care provider that would accept TRICARE compared with the 44 percent of nonenrolled beneficiaries who used a nonnetwork civilian primary care provider[26] (See Figure 5).

In addition, when compared with the results of the last survey (2008-2011), the percentages of nonenrolled beneficiaries who reported that they experienced problems finding a specialty care or mental health care provider increased in the most recent survey (2012-2015) for beneficiaries who used nonnetwork providers, but there were no changes over time if their specialty care or mental health care providers were in the network[27] (See Figure 6).

More Nonenrolled TRICARE Beneficiaries Reported Obtaining Appointments as Soon as Desired

Compared to the prior survey, a higher percentage of nonenrolled beneficiaries reported that they were able to obtain appointments as soon as they desired. Specifically, the percentage of nonenrolled beneficiaries who made non-urgent appointments for health care and reported that they were able to usually or always obtain an appointment as soon as they thought they needed increased from 87 percent in the 2008-2011 survey to 90 percent in the 2012-2015 survey.[28] However, the most commonly reported length of time they waited between making an appointment and actually seeing a provider did not change from the 2008-2011 surveys—most respondents in both surveys reported they were able to get appointments within 3 days (about 54 percent for both years' surveys).[29]

---

[26] The margins of error for the estimates of nonenrolled beneficiaries' problems finding civilian primary care provider (by network status) at the 95 percent confidence level are within plus or minus 5 percentage points. These estimates are significantly different from each other at the 95 percent confidence level.

[27] Changes over time for problems finding a primary care provider were not significant at the 95 percent confidence level. Twenty percent of nonenrolled beneficiaries with network primary care providers and 44 percent of those with nonnetwork primary care providers reported problems finding a primary care provider in the 2012-2015 survey.

[28] The margins of error for these estimates are within plus or minus 1 percentage point at the 95 percent confidence level. The difference in estimates is significant at the 95 percent confidence level.

[29] The margins of error for these estimates are within plus or minus 1 percentage point at the 95 percent confidence level. Respondents had the option of picking time frames for how long

The 2012-2015 survey also asked specific questions about how easy it was to get an appointment with specialty care providers and mental health care providers:[30]

- Of those nonenrolled beneficiaries who tried to make an appointment with a civilian specialty care provider, 84 percent reported it was "usually easy," or "always easy," to get appointments.[31] These results also varied by network status, as a higher percentage of those who used a network specialty care provider reported that they found it "usually easy" or "always easy" to get appointments (85 percent) compared to those that used a nonnetwork specialty care provider (74 percent).[32]
- Of those nonenrolled beneficiaries that received treatment or counseling from a civilian mental health care provider, 73 percent reported that when they needed treatment or counseling right away, they usually or always saw someone as soon as they wanted.[33] We found that this result did not change since the prior survey, nor did we find any statistically significant differences between beneficiaries' responses for seeing a network versus a nonnetwork mental health provider.

---

they had to wait, such as "same day," "1 day, or "2-3 days," all the way up to "31 days or longer."

[30] The survey asked this question for specialty care providers and for mental health care providers, but did not ask about the ease in obtaining primary care appointments.

[31] We could not compare this estimate to see how it has changed over time as the previous survey did not ask this question. The margin of error for this estimate is within plus or minus 1 percentage point at the 95 percent confidence level.

[32] The margins of error for these estimates are within plus or minus 7 percentage points at the 95 percent confidence level. The difference in estimates is significant at the 95 percent confidence level.

[33] The margin of error for this estimate is within plus or minus 10 percentage points at the 95 percent confidence level.

NONENROLLED BENEFICIARIES' POSITIVE RATINGS OF TRICARE HAVE GENERALLY INCREASED OVER TIME AND VARY COMPARED TO OTHER FEDERAL HEALTH PLANS

Ratings of TRICARE over Time

Nonenrolled beneficiaries' positive ratings of TRICARE have generally increased since the previous survey. Specifically, over time, nonenrolled beneficiaries' positive ratings of five different categories related to TRICARE have either increased (primary care rating, specialty care rating, and health plan rating) or remained the same (mental health care rating and health care rating)[34] (See Figure 7).

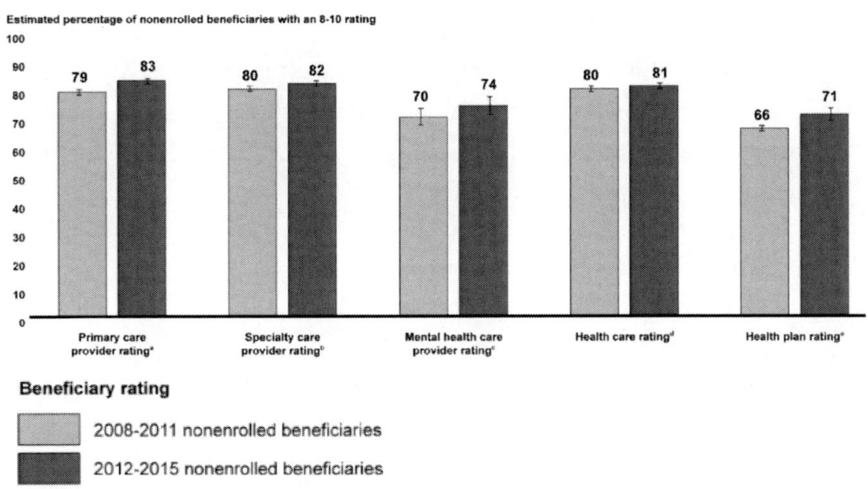

Source: GAO analysis of Department of Defense data. | GAO-18-361.

Notes: Percentages show the beneficiaries' reported ratings of 8-10 on a 0-10 scale. Bars display 95 percent confidence levels for estimates, rounded to a whole number.

Other than ratings of mental health care and health care, the differences in estimates between the 2008-2011 and the 2012-2015 survey results are statistically significant at the 95 percent confidence level.

[34] We refer to "positive ratings" as those nonenrolled beneficiaries rated their experiences between an 8 and a 10 on an ascending 0-10 scale for each of these categories.

[a]For the 2012-2015 survey, beneficiaries were asked "Using any number from 0 to 10, where 0 is the worst personal doctor possible, and 10 is the best personal doctor possible, what number would you use to rate your personal doctor?" The 2008-2011 survey question was the same, except it asked the beneficiary to rate the "personal doctor or nurse." Our analysis is limited to nonenrolled beneficiaries who indicated that their personal doctor was a civilian.

[b]Beneficiaries were asked "We want to know your rating of the specialist you saw most often in the last 12 months. Using any number from 0 to 10, where 0 is the worst specialist possible, and 10 is the best specialist possible, what number would you use to rate the specialist?" Our analysis is limited to nonenrolled beneficiaries who indicated that they had seen a civilian specialist in the last 12 months.

[c]Beneficiaries were asked "Using any number from 0 to 10, where 0 is the worst treatment or counseling possible, and 10 is the best treatment or counseling possible, what number would you use to rate all your treatment or counseling in the last 12 months?" Our analysis is limited to nonenrolled beneficiaries who indicated that they had seen a civilian mental health care provider.

[d]Beneficiaries were asked "Using any number from 0 to 10, where 0 is the worst health care possible, and 10 is the best health care possible, what number would you use to rate all your health care in the last 12 months?"

[e]Beneficiaries were asked "Using any number from 0 to 10, where 0 is the worst health plan possible, and 10 is the best health plan possible, what number would you use to rate your health plan?"

Figure 7. Comparison of Nonenrolled Beneficiaries' Estimated Positive Ratings of Their TRICARE Experiences, over Time.

Furthermore, nonenrolled beneficiaries' positive ratings of their mental health care providers were lower than their ratings for their primary and specialty care providers.

We also found that there were no significant differences at the 95 percent confidence level for nonenrolled beneficiaries' ratings of primary care, specialty care, or mental health care providers based on their network status.[35]

Ratings of TRICARE Compared to Other Federal Health Plans

When we compared these results to those of the 2013-2015 CAHPS surveys, we found that nonenrolled TRICARE beneficiaries' positive

---

[35] Due to the survey questions' wording for ratings with "health care" or "health plan," we could not analyze these ratings by the nonenrolled beneficiaries' reported providers' network status.

experience ratings for primary care providers and specialty care providers were lower than those of Medicare fee-for-service beneficiaries and higher than those of Medicaid beneficiaries, which is similar to what we found for the previous survey.[36] We also found that TRICARE beneficiaries' positive experience ratings for their health care were higher than that of both Medicare fee-for-service beneficiaries and Medicaid beneficiaries, but TRICARE beneficiaries' positive experience ratings for their health plan were lower than both of these groups (See Figure 8).

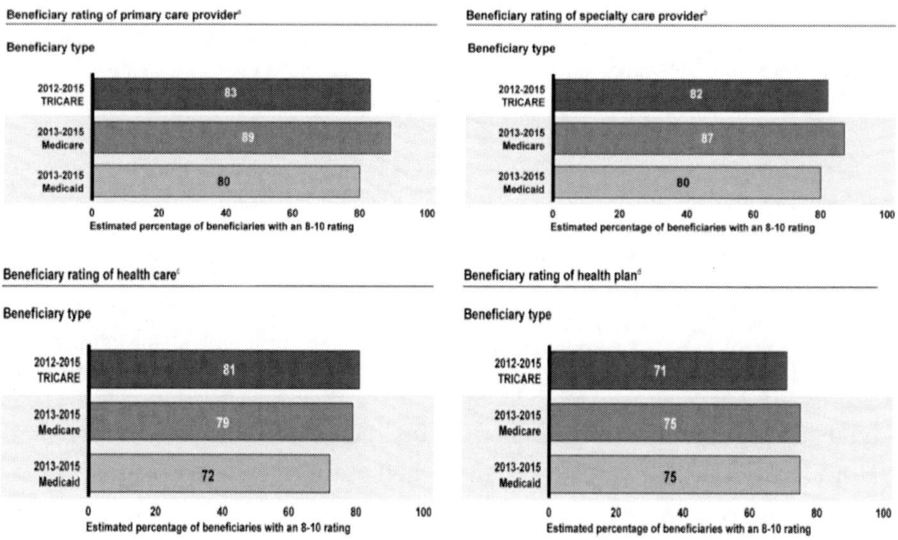

Source: GAO analysis of the Departments of Defense's and Health & Human Services' data. | GAO-18-361.

Notes: Percentages show the beneficiaries' reported ratings of 8-10 on a 0-10 scale.

For the 2012-2015 nonenrolled beneficiary survey, margins of error were within 2 percentage points for each rating estimate, at the 95 percent confidence level. For the 2013-2015 Medicare and Medicaid surveys, margins of error were within 0.3 percentage points for each rating estimate, at the 95 percent confidence level. Within rating categories, all differences in estimates between 2012-2015 nonenrolled beneficiary survey results and 2013-2015 Medicare and Medicaid beneficiaries' results are statistically significant at the 95 percent confidence level.

Estimates for Medicare and Medicaid beneficiaries are from the Department of Health and Human Services' 2013 through 2015 Consumer Assessment of Healthcare Providers and Systems

---

[36] We could not compare nonenrolled beneficiaries' positive ratings of their mental health care provider to those of Medicare or Medicaid beneficiaries, as the latter two surveys did not contain a relevant question. See GAO-13-364 for previous trends.

(CAHPS) surveys to Medicare and Medicaid beneficiaries. These surveys are administered to determine how beneficiaries rate their experiences in receiving care in the Medicare and Medicaid programs.

[a]Beneficiaries were asked "Using any number from 0 to 10, where 0 is the worst personal doctor possible, and 10 is the best personal doctor possible, what number would you use to rate your personal doctor?" Our analysis is limited to nonenrolled beneficiaries who indicated that their personal doctor was a civilian.

[b]TRICARE beneficiaries were asked "We want to know your rating of the specialist you saw most often in the last 12 months. Using any number from 0 to 10, where 0 is the worst specialist possible, and 10 is the best specialist possible, what number would you use to rate the specialist?" Medicare and Medicaid beneficiaries were asked the same question, but only in reference to the last 6 months. Our analysis is limited to nonenrolled beneficiaries who indicated that they had seen a civilian specialist in the last 12 months.

[c]TRICARE Beneficiaries were asked "Using any number from 0 to 10, where 0 is the worst health care possible, and 10 is the best health care possible, what number would you use to rate all your health care in the last 12 months?" Medicare and Medicaid beneficiaries were asked the same question, but only in reference to the last 6 months.

[d]Beneficiaries were asked "Using any number from 0 to 10, where 0 is the worst health plan possible, and 10 is the best health plan possible, what number would you use to rate your health plan?"

Figure 8. Nonenrolled TRICARE Beneficiaries' Estimated Experience Ratings Compared to Those of Medicare Fee-For-Service and Medicaid Beneficiaries.

Civilian Providers' Reported Awareness of TRICARE Has Generally Increased over Time, While Mental Health Providers' Acceptance of New TRICARE Patients Has Decreased

Civilian Providers' Awareness of TRICARE Has Generally Increased over Time, with Network Providers Reporting Higher Awareness than Nonnetwork Providers

Provider Awareness over Time, by Provider Type and by Location Type

Nationwide, a higher percentage of civilian providers reported that they were aware of TRICARE in the 2012-2015 civilian provider survey (84 percent) than those from the 2008-2011 civilian provider survey (82 percent).[37] Specifically, since the previous survey, we found that awareness increased for specialty care providers (from 92 to 94 percent) and mental health care providers (from 68 to 74 percent).[38]

In addition, when we analyzed these results by location type, we found that civilian providers in both PSAs and non-PSAs reported higher awareness of TRICARE since the previous survey (from 79 to 82 percent in PSAs and from 87 to 89 percent in non-PSAs).[39] Awareness among civilian providers in locations now designated as former PSAs remained statistically unchanged at the 95 percent confidence level (89 percent in 2012-2015). However, despite some increases in awareness, civilian providers in PSAs reported lower awareness than those in non-PSAs and former PSAs in the 2012-2015 surveys.[40]

Provider Awareness by Network Status

Providers within the TRICARE network reported higher awareness of TRICARE than nonnetwork providers, regardless of individual provider type (See Figure 9). Among individual provider types, the biggest difference in awareness between network and nonnetwork providers was for mental health care providers, with 96 percent of network mental health care providers reporting awareness of TRICARE compared with 72 percent of nonnetwork mental health care providers.[41]

---

[37] When rounded, the margins of error for civilian providers' awareness of TRICARE are within plus or minus 1 percentage point at the 95 percent confidence level. The difference in estimates is significant at the 95 percent confidence level.

[38] Awareness among primary care providers remained unchanged since the last survey. When rounded, the margins of error for the specialty care and mental health care providers' awareness of TRICARE are within plus or minus 2 percentage points at the 95 percent confidence level. Within each provider type, the differences in estimates are significant at the 95 percent confidence level.

[39] When rounded, the margins of error for civilian providers' awareness of TRICARE by location type are within plus or minus 1 percentage point at the 95 percent confidence level. Within each location type, the differences in estimates are significant at the 95 percent confidence level.

[40] We previously reported that civilian providers in PSAs had lower awareness of TRICARE than those in non-PSAs. See GAO-13-364.

[41] When rounded, the margins of error for mental health care providers' awareness of TRICARE are within plus or minus 2 percentage points at the 95 percent confidence level. The difference in estimates is significant at the 95 percent confidence level.

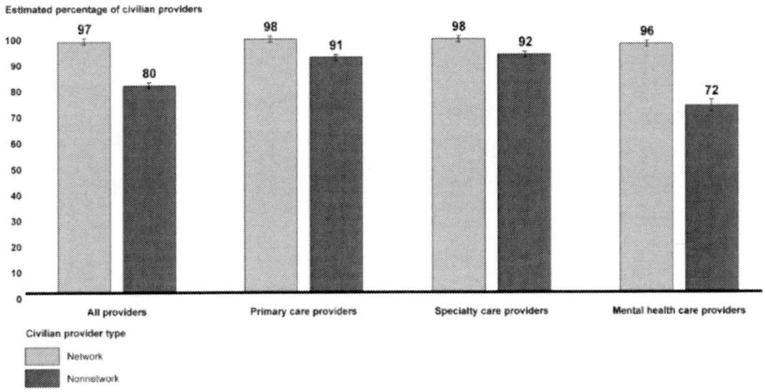

Source: GAO analysis of Department of Defense data. | GAO-18-361.

Notes: Bars display 95 percent confidence levels for estimates, rounded to a whole number. Within provider types, the differences between the network and nonnetwork providers are statistically significant at the 95 percent confidence level. Respondents answered "yes" to the survey question that asked "Is provider aware of the TRICARE health care program?"

Figure 9. Civilian Providers' Reported Awareness of TRICARE, by Provider Type and Network Status (2012-2015).

Civilian Mental Health Care Providers' Acceptance of New TRICARE Patients Has Decreased; Network Providers Reported Higher Acceptance than Nonnetwork Providers

Provider Acceptance over Time, by Provider Type and Location Type

Nationwide, we found an overall decrease reported in civilian providers' acceptance of new TRICARE patients in the 2012-2015 civilian provider survey (55 percent) compared to the 2008-2011 civilian provider survey (58 percent).[42]

However, when we analyzed acceptance by provider type, we found that the overall decrease was mainly attributable to a decrease in mental health

[42] When rounded, the margins of error for all civilian providers' acceptance of new TRICARE patients are within plus or minus 1 percentage point at the 95 percent confidence level. The difference in estimates is significant at the 95 percent confidence level.

care providers' acceptance rates, as primary and specialty care providers' acceptance rates remained unchanged.[43]

Of the 17 percent of network providers who reported that they were not accepting new TRICARE patients, some of the top reasons cited were

- not accepting any new patients,
- reimbursement, and
- do not know/no answer

Of the 53 percent of nonnetwork providers who reported that they were not accepting new TRICARE patients, some of the top reasons cited were

- not aware of TRICARE/Not asked/Don't know,
- miscellaneous, and
- specialty not covered

A Department of Defense official told us that some examples of "miscellaneous" are "in a private practice," and "not a preferred provider."

Source: GAO analysis of Department of Defense data. | GAO-18-361.

Specifically, mental health care providers' TRICARE acceptance rate decreased from 39 to 36 percent.[44] However, this low acceptance rate may not be an issue unique to TRICARE, as we have previously reported that there is a nationwide shortage of mental health professionals.[45]

In addition, when we analyzed results for all civilian providers by location type, we found that civilian providers in PSAs and non-PSAs

---

[43] Primary care providers' acceptance of new TRICARE patients was 67 percent in 2008-2011 and 68 in 2012-2015, and specialty care providers' acceptance of new TRICARE patients was 77 percent in 2008-2011 and 78 percent in 2012-2015. However, these differences for primary and specialty care were not statistically significant at the 95 percent confidence level.

[44] When rounded, the margins of error for civilian mental health providers' acceptance of new TRICARE patients are within plus or minus 1 percentage point at the 95 percent confidence level. The difference in estimates is significant at the 95 percent confidence level.

[45] See GAO, *VA Mental Health: Clearer Guidance on Access Policies and Wait-Time Data Needed,* GAO-16-24 (Washington, D.C.: Oct. 28, 2015).

reported lower acceptance rates of new TRICARE patients since the previous survey (from 55 to 53 percent in PSAs, and from 66 to 62 percent in non- PSAs).[46] Acceptance among civilian providers in locations now designated as former PSAs remained statistically unchanged at the 95 percent confidence level (60 percent in 2012-2015). Similar to our findings on providers' awareness, we found that civilian providers in PSAs reported lower acceptance rates than those in non-PSAs and former PSAs.[47]

Provider Acceptance by Network Status

When we analyzed civilian providers' acceptance of new TRICARE patients by providers' network status, we found that network providers reported higher acceptance of new TRICARE patients than nonnetwork providers, regardless of provider type (See Figure 10). Among individual provider types, the biggest difference in acceptance between network and nonnetwork providers was for mental health care providers with 79 percent of network mental health care providers reporting acceptance of new TRICARE patients compared with 30 percent of nonnetwork mental health care providers.[48] Of those mental health care providers that were not accepting new TRICARE patients, one of the top reasons reported by those not in the network was a lack of awareness of TRICARE.

Due to the relatively small number of network mental health providers who provided reasons for not accepting new TRICARE patients, it was not possible to identify one primary reason; however, some of the reasons they

---

[46] When rounded, the margins of error for civilian providers' acceptance of new TRICARE patients are within plus or minus 1 percentage point at the 95 percent confidence level. The difference in estimates is significant at the 95 percent confidence level. Acceptance rates of new TRICARE patients did not change for former PSAs.

[47] We previously reported that civilian providers in PSAs had lower awareness of TRICARE than those in non-PSAs. See GAO-13-364.

[48] When rounded, the margins of error for civilian mental health providers' acceptance of new TRICARE patients are within 3 percentage points at the 95 percent confidence level. The difference in estimates is significant at the 95 percent confidence level.

cited include reimbursement, not accepting new patients, and specialty was not covered.[49]

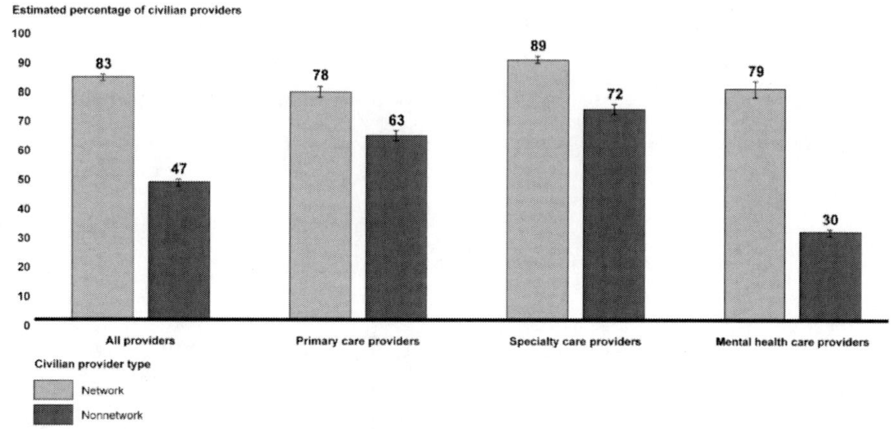

Source: GAO analysis of Department of Defense data. | GAO-18-361.

Notes: Bars display 95 percent confidence levels for estimates, rounded to a whole number.

Within provider types, the differences between the network and nonnetwork providers are statistically significant at the 95 percent confidence level.

Respondents answered "for all claims" or on a "claim-by-claim basis" to the survey question that asked "As of today, is the provider accepting new TRICARE Standard patients?"

Figure 10. Civilian Providers' Reported Acceptance of New TRICARE Patients, by Provider Type and Network Status (2012-2015).

DOD's Surveys of Nonenrolled Beneficiaries and Civilian Providers Collectively Indicate That Specific Geographic Locations May Have Access Problems

Our analysis of the 2012-2015 nonenrolled beneficiary and civilian provider surveys indicated that beneficiaries may have difficulty accessing a primary care provider, a specialty care provider, or both in 6 out of the 190

[49] The relatively low number of responses that provided reasons for why they were not accepting new TRICARE patients resulted in large margins of error.

specific geographic locations that were surveyed. For the 6 locations we identified, beneficiaries reported higher levels of problems finding providers, and providers reported lower rates of accepting TRICARE patients.[50]

- Primary care. We identified two locations where access to primary care providers may be particularly problematic (See Table 2). In these two locations, the percent of beneficiaries who reported that they had problems finding a primary care provider was at or above the 2012-2015 beneficiary survey's national average of 22 percent, and also where the percent of primary care providers who reported that they were accepting new TRICARE patients was at or below the 2012-2015 civilian provider survey's national average of 68 percent.[51]
- Specialty care. We identified five locations where access to specialty care providers may be particularly problematic (See Table 2). In these five locations, the percent of beneficiaries who reported that they had problems finding a specialty care provider was at or above the 2012-2015 beneficiary surveys' national average of 23 percent, and also where the percent of specialty care providers who reported that they were accepting new TRICARE patients was at or below the 2012-2015 civilian provider surveys' national average of 78 percent.[52]

---

[50] Because of the low numbers of survey responses for beneficiaries who said they needed civilian mental health care and responded to the question about whether they had a problem finding a civilian mental health care, we are unable to report correlated survey results for access problems to civilian mental health care providers.

[51] We excluded any individual locations that had less than (1) 30 respondents to the nonenrolled beneficiary survey questions about difficulties finding a specific type of provider, or (2) 50 respondents to the civilian providers' survey question about acceptance of new TRICARE surveys.

[52] We excluded any individual locations that had less than (1) 30 respondents to the nonenrolled beneficiary survey questions about difficulties finding a specific type of provider, or (2) 50 respondents to the civilian providers' survey question about acceptance of new TRICARE surveys.

When we compared this analysis to our analysis of the 2008-2011 beneficiary and provider surveys, the "Dallas/Fort Worth, Texas" HSA was identified in both results. Using data from the prior survey, our analysis identified it as being potentially problematic for primary care, but using data from the more recent survey, we identified specialty care access as being potentially problematic.[53] DOD officials told us that their past analysis of beneficiaries' complaints in this location centered on appointment wait times exceeding beneficiaries' preferences and on drive times to providers' offices. Officials explained that although there was a wide range of network specialty care providers in this location, TRICARE beneficiaries were a very small percentage of the overall population. Furthermore, this location is home to a number of large corporations that have health care plans that reimburse providers more than TRICARE. DOD officials added that due to these factors, providers in this location do not give preference to TRICARE beneficiaries, and drive times in this location are often long due to the traffic patterns and overall congestion of a large urban area.

Table 2. Locations with Both Potential Problems of Beneficiaries Not Finding Providers and Providers Not Accepting New TRICARE Patients, 2012-2015

Locations	Potential access problems with primary care[a]	Potential access problems with specialty care[b]
Prime Service Areas (PSAs)		
1. Bremerton/Seattle/Coupeville/Renton, Washington	✓	—
2. Brooklyn/Manhattan/Bronx/Jamaica, New York	✓	✓
3. Fort Worth/Dallas/Arlington/Denton, Texas	—	✓
4. Washington, DC/Rockville/Bethesda/Lanham, Maryland	—	✓
Former PSAs		
5. Dallas/McKinney/Amarillo/Rowlett, Texas	—	✓
Hospital Service Area (HSA)		
6. Dallas/Fort Worth, Texasc	—	✓

Source: GAO analysis of Department of Defense data. | GAO-18-361.

[53] See GAO-13-364.

Note: We included locations where the percentage of nonenrolled beneficiaries who experienced problems finding a civilian provider was at or above the 2012-2015 beneficiary surveys' national average and where the percentage of civilian providers who were accepting any new TRICARE patients was at or below the 2012-2015 civilian provider surveys' national average. Both determinations were made using the estimates' margins of error at the 95 percent confidence level. We identified and excluded any areas that had fewer than 50 respondents for the civilian provider surveys or 30 respondents for the question nonenrolled beneficiary surveys.

[a]Inclusion in this category was based on (1) nonenrolled beneficiaries' responses of "a big problem" or "a small problem" to the question that asked "In the last 12 months, how much of a problem was it to find a personal doctor or nurse who would accept TRICARE?" and (2) civilian primary care providers' responses of "for all claims" or a "claim-by-claim basis" to the question that asked "As of today, is the provider accepting new TRICARE Standard patients?"

[b]Inclusion in this category was based on (1) nonenrolled beneficiaries' responses of "a big problem" or "a small problem" to the question that asked "In the last 12 months, how much of a problem was it to find a doctor with this specialty who would accept TRICARE?" and (2) civilian specialty care providers' responses of "for all claims" or a "claim-by-claim basis" to the question that asked "As of today, is the provider accepting new TRICARE Standard patients?"

[c]The Dallas/Fort Worth, Texas, HSA is part of both the Dallas/McKinney/Amarillo/Rowlett, Texas Former PSA and the Fort Worth/Dallas /Arlington/Denton, Texas PSA.

AGENCY COMMENTS

In reviewing a draft of this chapter, DOD concurred with our overall findings. DOD's written response is reprinted in appendix I.

Debra A. Draper
Director
Health Care

APPENDIX I: COMMENTS FROM THE DEPARTMENT OF DEFENSE

THE ASSISTANT SECRETARY OF DEFENSE

1200 DEFENSE PENTAGON
WASHINGTON, DC 20301-1200

HEALTH AFFAIRS

MAR 15 2018

Ms. Debra A. Draper
Director, Health Care
U.S. Government Accountability Office
441 G. Street, N.W.
Washington, DC 20548

Dear Ms. Draper:

This is the Department of Defense response to the Government Accountability Office (GAO) Draft Report, GAO-18-361, "Defense Health Care: TRICARE Surveys Indicate Non-Enrolled Beneficiaries' Access to Care Has Generally Improved." Thank you for the opportunity to review and comment on the draft report.

Overall, I concur with the draft report's findings and conclusion. The report does not contain any recommendation, and I have no significant technical changes to offer, other than what we have provided to the analysts.

Sincerely,

for Tom McCaffery
Acting

In: Defense Health Care
Editor: Frederick Duncan

ISBN: 978-1-53615-175-6

Chapter 5

DEFENSE HEALTH CARE: TRICARE SELECT IMPLEMENTATION PLAN INCLUDED MANDATED ELEMENTS, BUT ACCESS STANDARDS SHOULD BE CLARIFIED*

United States Government Accountability Office

ABBREVIATIONS

DHA	Defense Health Agency
DOD	Department of Defense
MTF	military treatment facility
NDAA 2017	National Defense Authorization Act for Fiscal Year 2017

* This is an edited, reformatted and augmented version of the United States Government Accountability Office Report to Congressional Committees, Publication No. GAO-18-358, dated April 2018.

WHY GAO DID THIS STUDY

DOD offers health care services to approximately 9.4 million eligible beneficiaries through TRICARE, DOD's regionally structured health care program. In each of its regions, DOD uses contractors to manage health care delivery through civilian provider networks, among other tasks.

The NDAA 2017 made several changes to the TRICARE program, including the establishment of a new preferred provider network health plan option called TRICARE Select. The NDAA 2017 also required DOD to develop an implementation plan for TRICARE Select that addresses seven specific mandated elements on access to care, beneficiary complaints, and quality metrics for network providers.

The NDAA 2017 included a provision for GAO to review the implementation plan. This chapter examines the extent to which DOD's implementation plan addressed the mandated elements. GAO evaluated DOD's implementation plan using leading planning practices identified in GAO's prior work and standards for internal control. GAO examined program policies, procedures, and contracts and interviewed DOD officials and TRICARE regional contractors.

WHAT GAO RECOMMENDS

GAO recommends that DOD provide written documentation of its approach for developing and approving the TRICARE Select access standards, as well as the final access standards, to Congress. DOD agreed with GAO's recommendation.

WHAT GAO FOUND

The Department of Defense's (DOD) TRICARE Select Implementation Plan addressed the seven specific elements mandated by the National

Defense Authorization Act for Fiscal Year 2017 (NDAA 2017). These elements are

- Element A: ensuring that at least 85 percent of the TRICARE Select beneficiary population is covered by the network by January 1, 2018;
- Element B: ensuring access standards for health care appointments;
- Element C: establishing mechanisms for monitoring compliance with standards for access to care;
- Element D: establishing health care provider-to-beneficiary ratios;
- Element E: monitoring complaints by beneficiaries with respect to network adequacy and health care provider availability;
- Element F: establishing requirements for mechanisms to monitor the responses to complaints by beneficiaries; and
- Element G: establishing mechanisms to evaluate the quality metrics of the network providers.

GAO also assessed the implementation plan against leading practices for sound strategic management planning and found that it incorporated many of the practices, such as establishing goals, strategies to achieve goals, and plans to assess progress. However, a few of the leading practices were only partially incorporated or not incorporated at all. For example, the implementation plan did not always fully address the leading practice that planning documents include strategies to achieve goals and plans to assess progress. DOD officials explained that some of the details of their approach to the elements had not been finalized when they were completing the implementation plan. These officials added that their approach to the implementation plan was to create a strategic overview, and that some of the details are contained in contract documents and monitored through their oversight responsibilities.

Furthermore, GAO's assessment of the plan's elements found that the approach outlined in the implementation plan for ensuring access standards for health care appointments (Element B) is different from the approach DOD intends to use. The plan noted that DOD will use the access standards for TRICARE Prime—a managed care option—for TRICARE Select. However, DOD officials told GAO that the contractors are responsible for developing their own access standards, which DOD must approve. These officials added that DOD did not include information about the contractors proposing their own access standards because DOD was still developing its approach to this element when the plan was submitted. Because the implementation plan does not reflect DOD's current approach, Congress may not have the information it needs about the contractors' responsibilities for providing access to care, impeding its ability to provide oversight.

* * *

April 13, 2018

The Honorable John McCain
Chairman

The Honorable Jack Reed
Ranking Member
Committee on Armed Services
United States Senate

The Honorable Mac Thornberry
Chairman

The Honorable Adam Smith
Ranking Member
Committee on Armed Services
House of Representatives

In fiscal year 2017, the Department of Defense (DOD) offered health care services to over 9 million beneficiaries in the United States and abroad through TRICARE, DOD's regionally structured health care program.[1] In the past, beneficiaries had their choice of coverage among TRICARE's three basic health plan options—TRICARE Prime, a managed care option; TRICARE Standard, a fee-for service option; and TRICARE Extra, a preferred provider organization option.[2] The National Defense Authorization Act for Fiscal Year 2017 (NDAA 2017) required DOD to terminate two of these options, TRICARE Standard and Extra, and establish a new self-managed preferred provider option called TRICARE Select no later than January 1, 2018.[3] According to DOD, this change will modernize the TRICARE benefit—specifically by introducing a progressive health plan model with enrollment requirements for beneficiaries. It is also intended to improve beneficiaries' access to care—an issue we have previously reported on for beneficiaries who used the TRICARE Standard and Extra options.[4]

The NDAA 2017 also required DOD to develop an implementation plan for TRICARE Select that includes seven specifically defined elements on access to care, including elements related to TRICARE Select's network coverage, access standards for health care appointments, beneficiary complaints about network coverage and access, and quality metrics for

---

[1] Generally, TRICARE beneficiaries include active duty personnel and their dependents, National Guard and Reserve servicemembers and their dependents, and retirees and their dependents or survivors. Active duty personnel include Reserve component members on active duty for at least 30 days.

[2] Active duty servicemembers are required to use TRICARE Prime. TRICARE offers several other plans, including TRICARE Reserve Select (for certain Reserve servicemembers and their dependents), TRICARE Retired Reserve (for certain retired Reserve servicemembers and their families), and TRICARE Young Adult (Prime and Select options, for servicemembers' dependents who are at least age 21 but not yet 26 years old). TRICARE also offers TRICARE for Life to TRICARE beneficiaries who are eligible for Medicare and enroll in Part B. Under TRICARE for Life, TRICARE processes claims after they have been adjudicated by Medicare.

[3] Pub. L. No 114-328, §§ 701(a)(1) and (c), 130 Stat. 2000, 2180, 2187 (2016).

[4] For example, see GAO, Defense Health Care: More-Specific Guidance Needed for Assessing Nonenrolled TRICARE Beneficiaries' Access to Care, GAO-14-384 (Washington, D.C.: Apr. 28, 2014); Defense Health Care: TRICARE Multiyear Surveys Indicate Problems with Access to Care for Nonenrolled Beneficiaries, GAO-13-364 (Washington, D.C.: Apr. 2, 2013); and Defense Health Care: Access to Civilian Providers under TRICARE Standard and Extra, GAO-11-500 (Washington, D.C.: June 2, 2011).

providers.[5] DOD submitted this plan to Congress on August 7, 2017. The NDAA 2017 included a provision for us to review the adequacy of the plan in addressing the mandated elements.[6] In this chapter, we examine the extent to which DOD's implementation plan for TRICARE Select addressed these elements.

To conduct this assessment, we reviewed DOD's implementation plan, TRICARE program policies and procedures, and contract documents that require specific access-related plans and data reports from the contractors. We compared this information with the plan elements mandated by the NDAA 2017, leading practices for strategic management planning identified by our prior work, and standards for internal controls in the federal government.[7] (See app. I.) We also interviewed DOD officials, including officials from the Defense Health Agency (DHA), which oversees the TRICARE program, and the TRICARE Regional Offices, which oversee health care delivery in each TRICARE region, to understand the development and function of the plan, as well as the planned approach to addressing each element. We also interviewed representatives of the managed care support contractors, which manage health care delivery through civilian provider networks in each region, among other tasks, to understand any challenges related to implementation of the mandated elements.

We conducted this performance audit from July 2017 to April 2018 in accordance with generally accepted government auditing standards. Those standards require that we plan and perform the audit to obtain sufficient,

---

[5] Pub. L. No. 114-328, § 701(c), 130 Stat. at 2187-2188. The NDAA 2017 also included two additional implementation plan elements that were to be included if necessary or appropriate: (1) making recommendations for legislative action to carry out the plan, as necessary, and (2) any other element determined to be appropriate. Because these two elements were not addressed in DOD's implementation plan, we did not include them in the scope of our review.

[6] Pub. L. No 114-328, § 701(c), 130 Stat. at 2188.

[7] For an example of our prior work, see GAO, Military Readiness: DOD Needs to Incorporate Elements of a Strategic Management Planning Framework into Retrograde and Reset Guidance, GAO-16-414 (Washington, D.C.: May 13, 2016). Also, see GAO, Standards for Internal Control in the Federal Government, GAO-14-704G (Washington, D.C.: September 2014). Internal control is a process effected by an entity's management, oversight body, and other personnel that provides reasonable assurance that the objectives of an entity will be achieved.

appropriate evidence to provide a reasonable basis for our findings and conclusions based on our audit objectives. We believe that the evidence obtained provides a reasonable basis for our findings and conclusions based on our audit objectives.

BACKGROUND

TRICARE Regional Structure and Contracts

Under TRICARE, beneficiaries may obtain health care through DOD's system of military hospitals and clinics, referred to as military treatment facilities (MTF), or from civilian providers. DHA uses managed care support contractors to develop networks of civilian providers, referred to as network providers, to serve all TRICARE beneficiaries in geographic areas called Prime Service Areas.[8] The contractors also perform other customer service functions, such as processing claims and assisting beneficiaries with finding providers. Each TRICARE region within the United States has a managed care support contractor. In July 2016, DOD awarded its fourth generation of TRICARE managed care support contracts. The new contracts reduced the number of TRICARE regions from three (North, South, and West) to two (East and West).[9] On January 1, 2018, the TRICARE program began health care delivery under these contracts.

TRICARE's Health Plan Options

Prior to January 1, 2018, TRICARE's non-Medicare-eligible beneficiary population could obtain care through three basic health plan

[8] Prime Service Areas are geographic areas determined by the Assistant Secretary of Defense for Health Affairs and are usually within an approximate 40-mile radius of an MTF and at all Base Realignment and Closure sites, which are military installations that have been closed or realigned as a result of decisions made by the Commission on Base Realignment and Closure.

[9] The East region resulted from the merger of the North and South regions.

options— TRICARE Prime (managed care), TRICARE Standard (fee-for-service), and TRICARE Extra (preferred provider organization)—that varied by enrollment requirements, choices in civilian providers, and whether there were established access standards.[10] Beginning January 1, 2018, the TRICARE Standard and Extra options were terminated and TRICARE Select, a self-managed, preferred provider option, was established. (See table 1.)

Table 1. Summary of Selected Past and Current TRICARE Options

TRICARE option	Description of option
TRICARE Prime	• This managed care option requires enrollment.[a] • There is no enrollment fee for active duty servicemembers and their families, but most other beneficiaries must pay an annual enrollment fee. • Active duty servicemembers are required to use TRICARE Prime, while other beneficiaries have a choice. • Enrollees obtain most of their care from providers at military treatment facilities (MTF) but also may obtain care from TRICARE's network of civilian providers (network providers). • There are established access standards for this option.[b]
TRICARE Standard and TRICARE Extra (Terminated on January 1, 2018)	• These options did not require enrollment. • Beneficiaries could obtain health care from nonnetwork providers under TRICARE Standard,the fee-for-service option. • Beneficiaries could also choose to obtain care from network civilian providers under TRICARE Extra, the preferred provider option. • Beneficiaries were also able to receive care from MTFs, though they had a lower priority for receiving care than TRICARE Prime beneficiaries.

[10] The TRICARE non-Medicare-eligible beneficiary population includes all beneficiaries— such as active duty personnel and their dependents, National Guard and Reserve servicemembers and their dependents, and retired servicemembers and their dependents or survivors—who do not meet the requirements for obtaining health care coverage under Medicare. Medicare is available, generally, to people age 65 or older, younger people with disabilities, and people with end-stage renal disease.

TRICARE option	Description of option
	• There were no established access standards for these options.
TRICARE Select (Established on January 1, 2018)	• This self-managed, preferred provider option requires enrollment.[a] • There is no enrollment fee for active duty servicemembers and their families, but most otherbeneficiaries must pay an annual enrollment fee.[c] • Beneficiaries are able to obtain health care from network and nonnetwork providers.[d] • Beneficiaries are also able to receive care from MTFs, though they have a lower priority for receiving care than TRICARE Prime beneficiaries. • Access standards are required for this option.

Source: GAO summary of TRICARE program information. | GAO-18-358.

[a] Prior to January 1, 2019, beneficiaries are able to change plans at any time. On or after January 1, 2019, beneficiaries will only be able to change plans during an annual open enrollment season or within a certain time period following a qualifying life event. Qualifying life events include military changes—such as activating or deactivating, deploying, separating from active duty, or retiring—and family events—such as getting married or divorced, having or adopting a baby, becoming Medicare-eligible, or experiencing a death in the family. In general, beneficiaries are able to make enrollment changes within 90 days of such an event.

[b] The TRICARE Prime option has five access standards that set requirements for the following: (1) travel time to provider sites, (2) appointment wait time, (3) availability and accessibility of emergency services, (4) composition of network specialists, and (5) office wait time. See 32 C.F.R. § 199.17(p)(5) (2017).

[c] The amount of this enrollment fee is based upon a sponsor's initial enlistment date, among other factors.

[d] Nonnetwork providers are those providers that are not in the TRICARE network, but are certified to see TRICARE patients.

Beneficiaries using the TRICARE Standard and Extra options as of December 31, 2017, were automatically enrolled in TRICARE Select on January 1, 2018. Beneficiaries are allowed to change their plan at any time prior to January 1, 2019, after which they will only be able to change plans during an annual open enrollment season or within a certain time period following a qualifying life event.[11] In August 2017, DOD estimated that over

[11] Qualifying life events include military changes—such as activating or deactivating, deploying, separating from active duty, or retiring—and family events, such as getting married or divorced, having or adopting a baby, becoming Medicare-eligible, or experiencing a death in

2 million beneficiaries will be enrolled in TRICARE Select, which is approximately the same number of beneficiaries who used the TRICARE Standard option. According to DOD, approximately 66 percent of these beneficiaries resided in a Prime Service Area—where networks of civilian providers have been established.

TRICARE Select Implementation Plan

In addition to establishing the TRICARE Select option and making other TRICARE program changes, the NDAA 2017 required DOD to develop an implementation plan for TRICARE Select that includes seven specific elements. These elements are, in part, intended to ensure beneficiaries' access to care under the TRICARE Select option, and they require DOD to

- ensure that at least 85 percent of the beneficiary population under TRICARE Select is covered by the network by January 1, 2018 (Element A);
- ensure access standards for appointments for health care that meet or exceed those of high-performing health care systems in the United States, as determined by the Secretary (Element B);
- establish mechanisms for monitoring compliance with access standards (Element C);
- establish health care provider-to-beneficiary ratios (Element D);
- monitor on a monthly basis complaints by beneficiaries with respect to network adequacy and the availability of health care providers (Element E);
- establish requirements for mechanisms to monitor the responses to complaints by beneficiaries (Element F); and

---

the family. In general, beneficiaries are able to make enrollment changes within 90 days of such an event.

- establish mechanisms to evaluate the quality metrics of the network providers established under section 728 (of the NDAA 2017) (Element G).[12]

DOD'S TRICARE SELECT IMPLEMENTATION PLAN INCLUDED THE MANDATED ELEMENTS AND ADDRESSED MOST LEADING PLANNING PRACTICES, BUT DOES NOT REFLECT CURRENT APPROACH FOR ACCESS STANDARDS

DOD's Implementation Plan Included the Mandated Elements and Addressed Most Leading Practices for Strategic Management Planning

The TRICARE Select implementation plan DOD submitted to Congress included the seven specific elements mandated by the NDAA 2017. Specifically, the implementation plan described the upcoming changes to the TRICARE benefit and included individual sections outlining DOD's approach for implementing each of the required elements. For example, for element A—ensure that at least 85 percent of the beneficiary population under TRICARE Select is covered by the network by January 1, 2018—DOD described, among other things, how the regional contractors will identify geographic areas with concentrations of TRICARE Select beneficiaries and how they will establish a sufficient provider network to serve that population.

We also found that the implementation plan reflected most of the leading practices for sound strategic management planning as identified by our prior

---

[12] Section 728 of the NDAA 2017 requires that DOD, to the extent appropriate, adopt the core quality performance metrics agreed upon by the Core Quality Measures Collaborative, which comprises officials from the Centers for Medicare & Medicaid Services and representatives of health care organizations such as America's Health Insurance Plans, for use by the military health system and in contracts awarded to carry out the TRICARE program. Pub. L. No. 114-328, § 728(a)(1), 130 Stat. at 2233.

work.[13] (See table 2.) These leading practices suggest that strategic planning documents include the following: (1) a mission statement, (2) goals, (3) strategies to achieve goals, (4) plans to assess progress, and (5) identification of challenges and risks. For example, DOD's implementation plan clearly articulated a mission statement, which is "to ensure beneficiaries receive the right level of care, at the right time, delivered by the right provider."[14] Additionally, for six of the mandated elements, DOD's implementation plan outlined the goal, strategies to achieve the goal, and how DOD will assess progress. (See elements A, B, C, D, E, and F in table 2.) This information is supplemented by contract documents that require specific plans and data reports from the managed care support contractors. For example, for element A—ensure that at least 85 percent of the beneficiary population is covered by the network— each managed care support contractor is required to submit monthly performance reports that show that a sufficient number of providers in primary and specialty care are available to meet access requirements. While DOD's implementation plan addressed many of our leading practices, there were instances where some of the leading practices were only partially addressed or not addressed at all. For example, none of the mandated elements incorporated the leading practice related to identifying the challenges and risks that could affect the success of the element.

---

[13] GAO, Military Readiness: DOD Needs to Incorporate Elements of a Strategic Management Planning Framework into Retrograde and Reset Guidance, GAO-16-414 (Washington, D.C.: May 13, 2016). See app. I for a listing of GAO's leading practices for strategic management planning. For the purposes of this report, we combined the practices "use of metrics to gauge progress" and "evaluations of the plan to monitor goals and objectives" into a single category, referred to as "plans to assess progress" and renamed the practice "external factors that could affect goals" to "challenges and risks."

[14] For the purposes of this report, we evaluated whether a mission statement existed for the entire implementation plan rather than for each element.

Table 2. Extent to Which the Department of Defense's (DOD) August 2017 TRICARE Select Implementation Plan Addressed Select Leading Practices for Sound Strategic Management Planning

National Defense Authorization Act for Fiscal Year 2017 (NDAA 2017) mandated elements	Select leading practices for planning			
	Goals	Strategies to achieve goals	Plans to assess progress	Challenges and risks
Element A: Ensure that at least 85 percent of the beneficiary population under TRICARE Select is covered by the network by January 1, 2018	●	●	●	○
Element B: Ensure access standards for appointments for health care that meet or exceed those of high-performing health care systems in the United States, as determined by the Secretary	●	●	●	○
Element C: Establish mechanisms for monitoring compliance with access standards	●	●	●	○
Element D: Establish health care provider-to-beneficiary ratios	●	●	●	○
Element E: Monitor on a monthly basis complaints by beneficiaries with respect to network adequacy and the availability of health care providers	●	●	●	○
Element F: Establish requirements for mechanisms to monitor the responses to complaints by beneficiaries	●	●	●	○
Element G: Establish mechanisms to evaluate the quality metrics of the network providers established under section 728a	●	◐	○	○

Legend: ● Fully addressed practice ◐ Partially addressed practice ○ Did not address practice.

Source: GAO analysis of DOD's TRICARE Select implementation plan and supporting documentation. | GAO-18-358.

[a] Section 728 of the NDAA 2017 requires that DOD, to the extent appropriate, adopt the core quality performance metrics agreed upon by the Core Quality Measures Collaborative, which comprises officials from the Centers for Medicare & Medicaid Services and representatives of health care organizations such as America's Health Insurance Plans, for use by the military health system and in contracts awarded to carry out the TRICARE program.

Element G, Evaluation of Quality Metrics, Remains under Development

We also found that the implementation plan partially addressed or did not address the leading practices related to strategies or plans to assess progress for element G—establish mechanisms to evaluate the quality metrics of the network providers. The plan stated that DOD is reviewing the required set of core quality performance metrics and will implement a subset of these performance measures that can be used in future contracts. However, the plan did not include several strategic details such as (1) the process that DOD will use to determine the metrics, (2) the criteria and resources that are needed to select the subset of these performance measures, and (3) how DOD will assess progress and evaluate future metrics. DOD officials told us that a workgroup of departmental officials—including those from DHA and the TRICARE Regional Offices and representatives of the military service branches— with expertise in health care quality are

- evaluating the metrics for inclusion in the subset of measures based on criteria such as availability of data, the size of the population affected, and resources needed;
- developing a work plan and time frames to analyze the metrics that are (1) already being reported, (2) not being reported but data are available, and (3) not being reported and require data solutions in order to track information; and
- making preliminary recommendations on which measures to adopt and which to consider for future adoption.

DOD officials explained that some of the details of their approach to the mandated elements had not been finalized when they were completing the implementation plan, including some of the details for element G, which continues to be a work in progress. They added that they were under tight time constraints with competing priorities. They explained that they had to plan for the implementation of TRICARE Select while concurrently transitioning to new managed care support contracts, which had to be modified to incorporate this new health plan option.[15] Therefore, while DOD officials were developing the TRICARE Select implementation plan, they had to determine the specific program requirements for this option and modify the contracts to account for these changes.

Leading Practice on Challenges and Risks May Be Captured through Contract Oversight Mechanisms

We also found that DOD's implementation plan did not address the leading practice related to recognizing the challenges or risks to success for any of the seven elements. This practice ensures that an organization considers any external factors that could significantly affect the achievement of its goal. For example, for element A—ensure that at least 85 percent of the beneficiary population is covered by the network—the implementation plan did not address what challenges and risks the contractors might experience in establishing this network. For example, one of the two managed care support contractors stated that it did not have data on the beneficiaries who had sought coverage under TRICARE Standard and Extra as these beneficiaries did not have to enroll in these health plan options. Thus, the contractor explained that it was difficult to establish a baseline for calculating the 85 percent network coverage required for TRICARE Select. The other managed care support contractor told us that specific challenges included negotiating provider discounts in certain areas, identifying which providers participated in the past, and balancing the composition of the network between primary and specialty care. However, DOD officials told us that they considered and planned for the challenges and risks associated with certain elements—including establishing a monitoring and remediation process to help ensure contractors meet the 85 percent network coverage requirement—even though this was not described in the plan.

---

[15] The NDAA 2017 was enacted in December 2016—after the contracts were awarded and the same month that DOD commenced the contractor transition period, according to DOD officials. DOD officials noted that the establishment of the TRICARE Select option had not been accounted for in DOD's original contract requirements or transition timeline. DOD moved the health care delivery start date under the new contracts from October 1, 2017, to January 1, 2018, to allow time for these changes to be made and to coincide with the TRICARE Select implementation date.

DOD officials explained that their approach to the implementation plan was to create a strategic overview rather than a detailed work plan. These officials also told us that details and time frames related to the mandated elements are captured in contract documents, such as those that establish the managed care support contractors' reporting and planning requirements. Although these contract documents do not specifically address challenges and risks for each element, officials stated that they have oversight mechanisms in place that allow them to address any challenges faced by these contractors, thereby mitigating any potential risks. For example, DHA officials told us that the managed care support contractors provide status updates on their network expansion progress at weekly transition meetings with DHA and at biweekly meetings with the TRICARE Regional Offices. DHA officials told us that the TRICARE contracts have specific expansion goals and deadlines, such as requiring that 50 percent of network providers are in the system 120 days prior to the start of health care delivery. Given that both TRICARE Select and the new TRICARE contracts were implemented on January 1, 2018, it is too early to determine whether this approach will be sufficient to deal with any upcoming challenges and risks.

Implementation Plan Does Not Reflect Current Approach for Establishing Access Standards

Our review of element B—ensure access standards for appointments for health care that meet or exceed those of high-performing health care systems in the United States, as determined by the Secretary—noted that the approach described in the implementation plan differs from the approach that DOD intends to use. The implementation plan states that the access standards for TRICARE Select will mirror those of TRICARE Prime, DOD's managed care option, and that DOD will continue to compare these standards with those of high-performing U.S. health care systems. However, DOD officials told us in interviews that the access standards for TRICARE Select will be developed by each managed care support contractor and approved by DOD. This approach is outlined in contract documents, which state that the contractors are required to develop access-to-care plans that detail how they will ensure access standards that meet or exceed those of high-performing health care systems in the United States. DOD officials told us that they did not intend to suggest in the plan that the TRICARE Prime access standards would be applied to TRICARE Select. Instead, these officials explained that they meant that the access standards for TRICARE Select would be evaluated with the same tools as the access standards for TRICARE Prime. DOD officials further stated that they did not include information about the managed care support contractors proposing their own access standards because they were still developing the approach to this element when the implementation plan was submitted. DOD officials told us they decided on this approach because there is no national model for preferred provider organization access standards, and therefore they did not want to be prescriptive about the access standards for this option. However, as a result of this approach, there is the potential that the managed care support contractors for the East and West regions could be using two different sets of access standards for TRICARE Select. Standards for internal control in the federal government state that management should externally communicate the necessary information to achieve the entity's objectives.[16] Because the implementation plan does not reflect DOD's current approach, Congress may be lacking important information, including what responsibilities the contractors have in terms of providing access to care, impeding its ability to provide oversight.

CONCLUSION

On January 1, 2018, DOD implemented significant changes to the TRICARE program, which provides health care to millions of beneficiaries worldwide. One of these changes is the establishment of a new preferred provider option—TRICARE Select—intended to modernize the TRICARE benefit and improve beneficiaries' access to care. While DOD's

---

[16] GAO-14-704G.

implementation plan for this new option addressed all of the elements that were required, time constraints along with competing priorities impeded DOD's ability to fully develop its approach for some elements, which are being addressed through other oversight efforts. Furthermore, although one of TRICARE Select's primary goals is to improve access to care, DOD's implementation plan does not reflect how access standards will be established. Without the most current information, it will be difficult for Congress to determine whether the department is achieving its mission of ensuring that beneficiaries receive the right level of care, at the right time, delivered by the right provider.

Recommendation for Executive Action

We recommend that the Secretary of Defense direct the Assistant Secretary of Defense (Health Affairs) to provide written documentation of DOD's approach to developing and approving the TRICARE Select access standards, as well as the final access standards, to Congress. (Recommendation 1)

Agency Comments

We provided a draft of this chapter to DOD for comment. In its written comments, which are reproduced in Appendix II, DOD concurred with our recommendation. DOD stated that it will provide written documentation about the TRICARE Select access standards to Congress by June 30, 2018. DOD did not provide technical comments.

Debra A. Draper
Director,
Health Care

APPENDIX I: LEADING PRACTICES FOR STRATEGIC MANAGEMENT PLANNING AS IDENTIFIED BY GAO'S PRIOR WORK

This appendix provides additional information regarding six elements identified by our prior work as leading practices for strategic management planning to establish a comprehensive, results-oriented framework. (See table 3.)

Table 3. Six Leading Practices for Strategic Management Planning Identified by GAO's Prior Work

Key leading practice	Description of leading practice components
Mission statement	A statement that concisely summarizes what the organization does, presenting the main purposes for all its major functions and operations.
Long-term goals	A specific set of policy, programmatic, and management goals for the programs and operations covered in the plan. The long-term goals should correspond to the purposes set forth in the mission statement and develop with greater specificity how an organization will carry out its mission.
Strategies to achieve goals	A description of how goals contained in the plan are to be achieved, including the operational processes, skills and technology, and other resources required to meet these goals.
Use of metrics to gauge progress	A set of metrics that will be applied to gauge progress toward attainment of the plan's long-term goals.
Evaluations of the plan to monitor goals and objectives	Assessments, through objective measurement and systematic analysis, of the manner and extent to which programs associated with the plan achieve their intended goals.
External factors that could affect goals	Key factors external to the organization and beyond its control that could significantly affect the achievement of the long-term goals contained in the plan. These external factors can include economic, demographic, social, technological, or environmental factors, as well as conditions or events that would affect the organization's ability to achieve its strategic goals.

Source: GAO. | GAO-18-358.

Note: Source is Military Readiness: DOD Needs to Incorporate Elements of a Strategic Management Planning Framework into Retrograde and Reset Guidance, GAO-16-414 (Washington, D.C.: May 13, 2016), 28.

APPENDIX II: COMMENTS FROM THE DEPARTMENT OF DEFENSE

THE ASSISTANT SECRETARY OF DEFENSE

1200 DEFENSE PENTAGON
WASHINGTON, DC 20301-1200

HEALTH AFFAIRS

APR - 3 2018

Ms. Debra Draper
Director, Health Care
U.S. Government Accountability Office
441 G Street, NW
Washington, DC 20548

Dear Ms. Draper:

This is the Department of Defense (DoD) response to the Government Accountability Office (GAO) Draft Report, GAO-18-358, "TRICARE Select Implementation Plan Included Mandated Elements, but Access Standard Should Be Clarified," dated February 22, 2018. Thank you for the opportunity to review and comment on the draft report.

I concur with your sole recommendation that the Secretary of Defense provide written documentation of its approach for developing and approving the TRICARE Select access standards, as well as the final access standards to Congress. We will provide written documentation to Congress by June 30, 2018.

Sincerely,

Tom McCaffery
Acting

INDEX

A

accountability, 7, 27, 34, 36, 41, 47, 133, 200
administrative support, 47, 52, 107
adverse effects, 31, 128
agencies, 50, 52, 65, 69, 91, 97, 99, 115, 118, 121, 128, 133, 141
Air Force, viii, 2, 8, 12, 19, 29, 48, 51, 58, 61, 64, 65, 66, 68, 72, 75, 80, 85, 87, 90, 95, 102, 103, 104, 109, 110, 115, 116, 117, 118, 119, 121, 122, 123, 124, 126, 131, 132, 135, 139
armed forces, 54, 60, 67, 77, 79
Army, viii, 2, 8, 12, 19, 29, 51, 58, 61, 64, 65, 66, 68, 72, 75, 79, 80, 85, 87, 90, 94, 95, 102, 103, 104, 109, 110, 111, 114, 115, 116, 117, 118, 119, 121, 124, 126, 132, 135, 139

B

budgetary resources, 123
business processes, 52, 60, 99

C

challenges, vii, ix, 21, 28, 70, 84, 86, 88, 89, 90, 91, 107, 108, 114, 117, 118, 119, 120, 122, 124, 126, 127, 128, 129, 130, 132, 133, 134, 138, 139, 140, 186, 192, 195, 196
civil service, 128
civil service reform, 128
civilian providers, vii, viii, ix, 2, 5, 9, 13, 16, 18, 20, 21, 22, 27, 30, 31, 34, 35, 146, 147, 149, 150, 151, 152, 153, 156, 157, 158, 159, 162, 163, 165, 171, 172, 173, 174, 175, 176, 177, 179, 185, 187, 188, 190
collaboration, 91, 133, 135, 141
colorectal cancer, 25
Congress, iv, vii, viii, 2, 6, 7, 9, 12, 21, 23, 24, 26, 27, 34, 45, 46, 47, 48, 50, 52, 53, 54, 58, 65, 72, 73, 88, 98, 100, 111, 127, 182, 184, 186, 191, 197, 198, 200
construction, 53, 56, 57, 58, 76, 88, 91, 100
coordination, 73, 74, 131, 135
core dashboard, viii, 2, 7, 14, 15, 18, 19, 21, 23, 24, 25, 26, 27, 28, 29, 30, 33, 35, 36, 38, 40

cost, viii, 6, 23, 44, 47, 52, 53, 60, 67, 70, 84, 85, 88, 89, 96, 97, 98, 101, 107, 109, 110, 111, 112, 113, 115, 122, 124, 131, 134, 135, 136, 138, 156
cost effectiveness, 110
cost saving, 47, 52, 67, 98, 107, 123, 131
counseling, 152, 161, 163, 164, 165, 167, 169
criminal investigations, 105

D

Defense Health Agency (DHA), viii, 1, 12, 13, 15, 28, 29, 38, 40, 41, 43, 44, 45, 46, 47, 48, 49, 50, 51, 52, 53, 54, 55, 56, 57, 58, 59, 60, 61, 62, 63, 64, 65, 66, 67, 68, 69, 70, 71, 72, 73, 74, 75, 76, 77, 78, 79, 80, 83, 85, 86, 88, 89, 91, 93, 96, 99, 100, 108, 114, 116, 117, 127, 128, 129, 130, 131, 133, 134, 135, 139, 140, 181, 186, 187, 194, 196
Department of Health and Human Services, 23, 145, 152, 170
deployments, 90, 103, 106, 108, 110, 130, 131, 137, 141
draft, x, 36, 47, 49, 54, 67, 74, 85, 136, 147, 179, 198

E

education, 77, 78, 85, 101, 110, 112, 113
emergency, 16, 17, 63, 95, 105, 189
emergency response, 63
employees, 54, 60, 67, 77, 97, 98, 105, 118, 120, 132
employers, 122
employment, 112, 118
enrollment, 29, 156, 157, 185, 188, 189, 190
environment, 39, 92, 107
environmental factors, 199
evacuation, 63, 94, 95, 102, 106
evidence, 6, 9, 10, 52, 92, 141, 154, 187
execution, 47, 56, 78, 85, 99, 100, 114, 128
expertise, 15, 38, 117, 194

F

families, viii, 44, 185, 188, 189
federal agency, 121
federal government, 9, 69, 88, 97, 113, 123, 124, 186, 197, 200
federal hiring, 118, 123
federal regulations, 128
fee- for-service, ix, 146
fiscal policy, 88
fiscal year, viii, ix, 2, 3, 5, 12, 15, 44, 47, 48, 53, 58, 61, 65, 84, 88, 90, 91, 93, 103, 106, 108, 110, 116, 117, 118, 122, 123, 125, 126, 132, 136, 137, 138, 139, 149, 154, 157, 158, 184
force, 40, 52, 92, 97, 100, 101, 108, 110, 112, 116, 125, 126, 132, 139
funding, 80, 103, 112, 200
funds, 12, 56, 61, 88, 99, 200

G

governance, vii, 8, 9, 15, 28, 36, 39, 45, 47, 52, 55, 57, 58
guidance, 39, 40, 41, 56, 69, 73, 74, 89, 90, 97, 98, 99, 101, 104, 105, 106, 112, 113, 115, 122, 136, 138, 139

H

Health and Human Services, 23, 40, 145, 152, 170
health care, viii, ix, x, 3, 5, 6, 7, 8, 10, 11, 12, 13, 14, 15, 16, 19, 21, 23, 24, 26, 27, 28, 33, 34, 44, 47, 48, 52, 53, 57, 58, 63, 64, 67, 68, 76, 77, 78, 79, 87, 88, 91, 92,

95, 96, 100, 107, 114, 118, 120, 121, 126, 127, 128, 129, 135, 140, 146, 147, 148, 149, 150, 152, 154, 156, 159, 162, 165, 166, 167, 168, 169, 170, 171, 172, 173, 174, 175, 177, 178, 182, 183, 184, 185, 186, 187, 188, 189, 190, 191, 193, 194, 195, 196, 197
health care costs, 88
health care programs, 12
health care system, 6, 16, 47, 53, 77, 88, 190, 193, 196
health information, 21
health insurance, 152
health plan, viii, x, 5, 14, 16, 17, 21, 22, 24, 26, 28, 147, 151, 152, 161, 162, 163, 164, 165, 168, 169, 170, 171, 182, 185, 187, 195
health services, 106
hiring, 86, 90, 100, 114, 117, 118, 119, 120, 123, 124, 126, 128, 130, 132, 139
House of Representatives, 5, 13, 29, 46, 49, 55, 87, 149, 184
human, 117, 118, 127, 128, 135, 140
human capital, 127, 128, 135, 140
human resources, 117, 118

I

information technology, 12, 21, 48, 53, 57, 58, 76, 78, 91, 100
integration, 52, 78, 99, 112, 135

L

labor market, 90, 139
leadership, 3, 6, 8, 21, 22, 24, 26, 27, 28, 34, 36, 39, 40, 60, 91, 117, 133, 134, 140, 141
legislation, 100
logistics, 63, 105, 106

M

managed care, ix, 12, 13, 14, 16, 20, 30, 31, 32, 34, 36, 40, 146, 149, 156, 157, 184, 185, 186, 187, 188, 192, 194, 195, 196
management, ix, 8, 9, 12, 14, 18, 27, 33, 40, 44, 47, 48, 49, 50, 52, 53, 56, 57, 58, 59, 61, 67, 68, 69, 70, 71, 74, 76, 77, 78, 86, 90, 91, 96, 97, 98, 99, 100, 114, 115, 117, 119, 122, 127, 128, 129, 131, 133, 134, 135, 139, 140, 183, 186, 191, 192, 197, 199
manpower, 69, 71, 72, 74, 89, 97, 98, 108, 114, 126, 137, 139
Marine Corps, 8, 12, 13, 48, 80, 87, 102
medical, vii, ix, 3, 5, 7, 8, 10, 12, 16, 17, 18, 23, 24, 25, 26, 31, 32, 35, 36, 38, 39, 40, 44, 45, 47, 48, 50, 52, 53, 54, 56, 57, 58, 59, 60, 62, 63, 71, 72, 73, 75, 76, 77, 78, 79, 80, 84, 85, 87, 88, 89, 90, 91, 92, 93, 94, 95, 96, 99, 100, 101, 102, 103, 104, 106, 107, 109, 110, 111, 112, 113, 114, 115, 116, 117, 118, 120, 121, 127, 129, 130, 131, 132, 134, 135, 136, 137, 138, 139, 141, 149
medical care, ix, 76, 84, 87, 90, 92, 93, 94, 95, 104, 106, 107, 108, 109, 129, 130, 134, 135, 137
medical personnel, vii, ix, 84, 85, 87, 89, 90, 92, 94, 96, 101, 102, 103, 104, 107, 109, 110, 111, 113, 114, 115, 117, 130, 132, 134, 135, 136, 138
Medicare, viii, x, 1, 2, 3, 7, 8, 16, 17, 18, 22, 23, 24, 26, 32, 35, 39, 47, 56, 88, 146, 147, 152, 155, 156, 159, 170, 171, 185, 187, 188, 189, 191, 193
mental health, ix, 15, 120, 146, 147, 148, 149, 150, 152, 153, 154, 159, 160, 162, 165, 166, 167, 168, 169, 170, 172, 173, 174, 175, 177

mental health care, ix, 146, 147, 148, 149, 150, 152, 154, 159, 162, 165, 166, 167, 168, 169, 170, 172, 173, 174, 175, 177
mental health professionals, 174
military health system, vii, viii, 1, 3, 4, 5, 13, 14, 21, 24, 26, 38, 44, 46, 47, 51, 52, 53, 54, 55, 56, 57, 58, 60, 64, 65, 67, 70, 78, 83, 86, 87, 132, 191, 193
military hospitals, viii, 2, 3, 12, 15, 48, 58, 65, 88, 149, 187
military treatment facilities (MTFs), v, vii, viii, ix, 5, 9, 12, 13, 14, 18, 19, 21, 24, 26, 27, 28, 29, 33, 35, 43, 44, 45, 46, 47, 48, 49, 50, 53, 54, 55, 57, 58, 60, 61, 66, 71, 72, 73, 74, 75, 84, 85, 86, 87, 89, 90, 91, 92, 93, 94, 95, 100, 114, 115, 116, 117, 118, 119, 120, 122, 123, 124, 125, 126, 127, 128, 129, 130, 131, 132, 133, 134, 135, 139, 140, 149, 156, 157, 158, 163, 187, 188, 189
mission, 12, 39, 51, 65, 68, 69, 72, 88, 89, 92, 96, 97, 102, 105, 108, 109, 112, 115, 122, 123, 129, 130, 134, 137, 192, 198, 199
missions, 62, 64, 68, 71, 74, 85, 87, 98, 102, 103, 105, 114, 129
models, 114
morale, 124
moratorium, 97, 98, 119

N

National Defense Authorization Act (NDAA), vii, viii, ix, x, 2, 3, 6, 7, 9, 12, 17, 18, 20, 22, 29, 33, 43, 44, 45, 47, 48, 49, 50, 53, 54, 55, 57, 62, 67, 69, 75, 84, 88, 91, 98, 100, 103, 127, 132, 138, 145, 146, 149, 150, 151, 156, 158, 159, 181, 182, 183, 185, 186, 190, 191, 193, 195
national security, 105
Navy, viii, 2, 8, 12, 13, 19, 29, 48, 51, 61, 64, 65, 66, 68, 72, 75, 80, 85, 87, 90, 95, 102, 103, 104, 109, 110, 114, 115, 116, 117, 118, 121, 122, 123, 124, 125, 132, 135, 139
nonenrolled beneficiaries, v, vii, ix, 145, 146, 147, 150, 151, 152, 153, 154, 155, 157, 158, 159, 162, 165, 166, 167, 168, 169, 170, 171, 176, 179, 185

O

occupational health, 45, 88
officials, viii, x, 2, 8, 9, 18, 21, 22, 25, 27, 28, 29, 30, 32, 33, 45, 47, 51, 64, 65, 66, 67, 69, 72, 85, 86, 89, 90, 91, 92, 98, 99, 102, 104, 106, 107, 109, 110, 114, 115, 117, 118, 119, 120, 121, 122, 123, 124, 125, 126, 127, 129, 130, 131, 132, 133, 137, 138, 139, 140, 146, 153, 157, 159, 162, 178, 182, 183, 184, 186, 191, 193, 194, 195, 196, 197
operations, 47, 50, 51, 58, 64, 66, 68, 78, 88, 91, 97, 98, 102, 105, 112, 123, 124, 125, 129, 130, 132, 140, 141, 199
opportunities, 10, 66, 73, 108, 130, 137
outpatient, 7, 8, 16, 17, 19, 22, 24, 26, 36, 41, 149, 157, 158, 163
oversight, 9, 47, 56, 58, 70, 71, 77, 99, 183, 184, 186, 196, 197, 198, 200

P

performance standards, vii, viii, 2, 3, 6, 7, 9, 27, 28, 29, 30, 31, 33, 35, 36, 41
personnel costs, 85, 88, 136
physicians, 5, 22, 87, 106, 108, 111, 120, 121, 125
policy, ix, 15, 53, 56, 57, 58, 68, 76, 77, 78, 84, 85, 88, 90, 91, 97, 100, 102, 105,

109, 111, 112, 113, 117, 122, 133, 139, 199, 200
population, 19, 20, 30, 32, 102, 114, 155, 178, 183, 187, 188, 190, 191, 192, 193, 194, 195
preferred provider organization, ix, 146, 150, 185, 188, 197
private insurers, viii, 2, 8, 35
private practice, 174
private sector, 41, 53, 86, 87, 89, 92, 97, 98, 108, 118, 120, 121, 122, 123, 125, 137
provider network, viii, x, 14, 31, 157, 158, 163, 164, 165, 182, 186, 191
public health, 55, 80
public interest, 97
purchased care dashboard, viii, 2, 4, 7, 9, 15, 18, 19, 20, 21, 22, 23, 24, 25, 26, 27, 30, 34, 35, 36, 38, 39, 40, 41

Q

quality control, 125
quality improvement, 7, 15, 17, 18, 27, 32, 34
quality of care, viii, 2, 3, 4, 5, 6, 7, 10, 16, 18, 19, 20, 21, 23, 24, 27, 29, 30, 31, 32, 33, 34, 40, 122
quality standards, 37, 42

R

recommendations, iv, 2, 35, 36, 44, 53, 56, 70, 71, 72, 73, 74, 85, 99, 134, 136, 186, 194, 200
recruiting, 78, 112, 120
reform, 47, 49, 50, 51, 53, 60, 73, 86, 91, 98, 100, 128, 134, 140
reforms, 50, 60
reliability, 63, 90, 91, 125, 137, 138, 139, 153, 200
remediation, 37, 195
reserves, 93
resources, 11, 56, 57, 65, 69, 99, 115, 117, 118, 123, 194, 199
response, vii, viii, 3, 6, 9, 14, 38, 44, 48, 63, 74, 103, 127, 138, 150, 151, 153, 179
risk management, 78

S

safety, 11, 16, 20, 29, 31, 78, 124
Secretary of Defense, 5, 12, 14, 35, 36, 38, 45, 47, 48, 50, 51, 54, 55, 56, 57, 58, 60, 61, 62, 63, 64, 65, 66, 67, 68, 69, 70, 71, 72, 73, 74, 75, 76, 77, 79, 83, 84, 90, 91, 96, 98, 99, 100, 118, 135, 137, 187, 198
security, 97, 105, 106
security services, 106
Senate, ix, 4, 13, 29, 46, 49, 55, 69, 84, 87, 88, 148, 184
servicemembers, 5, 44, 47, 64, 87, 94, 104, 149, 154, 156, 185, 188, 189
services, iv, x, 5, 8, 11, 12, 13, 14, 15, 19, 28, 29, 30, 33, 37, 52, 53, 64, 65, 69, 71, 72, 86, 87, 93, 95, 96, 100, 101, 106, 107, 115, 116, 119, 123, 124, 125, 126, 127, 128, 131, 135, 140, 149, 182, 184, 189
staffing, ix, 11, 12, 67, 76, 79, 84, 90, 100, 106, 125, 127, 130, 131, 139
strategic management, 183, 186, 191, 192, 199
strategic planning, 192
structure, vii, 12, 23, 32, 36, 39, 41, 45, 47, 52, 55, 57, 58, 74, 91, 101, 140
survivors, 5, 96, 149, 154, 185, 188

T

technical comments, 198
technology, 12, 21, 48, 53, 57, 58, 76, 78, 91, 100, 199

testing, 19, 20
time constraints, 72, 194, 198
time frame, 150, 166, 194, 196
training, 12, 64, 85, 89, 96, 107, 110, 111, 112, 115, 126, 138
treatment, 2, 5, 13, 21, 24, 26, 43, 45, 47, 48, 50, 54, 63, 75, 76, 77, 78, 79, 83, 87, 93, 94, 95, 116, 135, 139, 149, 152, 156, 157, 158, 161, 163, 164, 165, 167, 169, 181, 187, 188
TRICARE Extra, vii, ix, 146, 150, 151, 156, 185, 188
TRICARE Prime, ix, 146, 149, 156, 184, 185, 188, 189, 196

U

United States, v, vi, 1, 4, 13, 14, 16, 23, 29, 43, 46, 48, 49, 50, 53, 54, 55, 57, 58, 59, 60, 61, 65, 75, 83, 87, 92, 94, 95, 96, 116, 121, 124, 129, 145, 148, 149, 181, 184, 187, 190, 193, 196

W

workforce, vii, ix, 53, 55, 69, 70, 72, 76, 84, 85, 86, 87, 88, 89, 90, 92, 95, 96, 97, 98, 99, 100, 103, 104, 105, 106, 107, 108, 110, 113, 114, 115, 116, 117, 122, 123, 124, 127, 128, 131, 132, 134, 135, 136, 138, 139, 140, 141
workforce mix, vii, ix, 84, 85, 86, 88, 89, 90, 96, 98, 104, 106, 108, 114, 116, 117, 122, 128, 134, 136, 138, 139, 140
workload, 68, 108, 114, 130
worldwide, 88, 197

U.S. Health Care Workforce: Supply and Demand Projections and Federal Planning Efforts

Editor: Sheldon T. Barrett

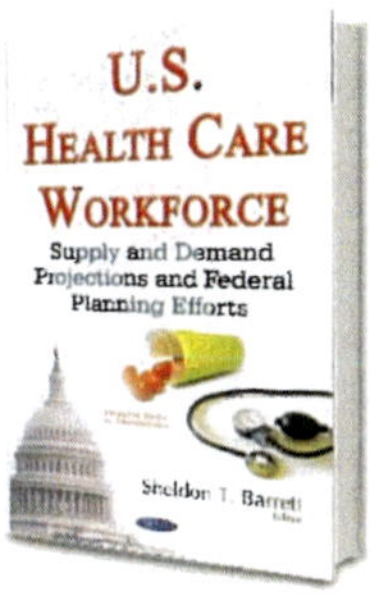

Series: Health Care in Transition

Book Description: This book provides a review on the supply and demand projections and federal planning efforts in the U.S. health care workforce.

Hardcover ISBN: 978-1-63485-730-7
Retail Price: $150

Health Care Use of Electronically Readable Cards: Prospects and Fraud Prevention Role

Editor: Rochelle Briggs

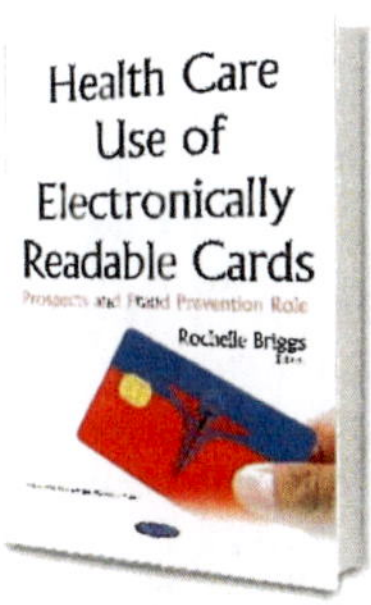

Series: Health Care in Transition

Book Description: Proposals have been put forward to replace the current paper Medicare cards, which display beneficiaries' Social Security numbers, with electronically readable cards, and to issue electronically readable cards to providers as well.

Softcover ISBN: 978-1-53610-116-4
Retail Price: $95

FUNDAMENTALS OF LEADERSHIP FOR HEALTHCARE PROFESSIONALS

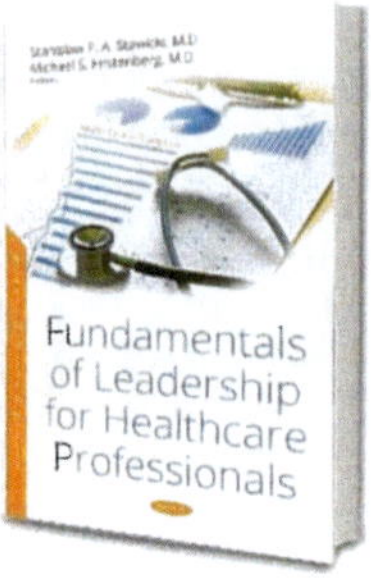

EDITORS: Stanislaw P. A. Stawicki, M.D. (Department of Research and Innovation, St Luke's University Health Network, Bethlehem, Pennsylvania, US); Michael S. Firstenberg, M.D. (Department of Surgery (Cardiothoracic), The Medical Center of Aurora, Aurora, Colorado, US)

SERIES: Health Care in Transition

BOOK DESCRIPTION: Each chapter in this text explores different aspects of healthcare leadership, provides valuable insights into how effective leadership functions, and offers practical perspectives on implementations of theory into practice.

HARDCOVER ISBN: 978-1-53613-620-3
RETAIL PRICE: $195

HEALTH INSURANCE: REQUIREMENTS, CHALLENGES, AND REGULATIONS

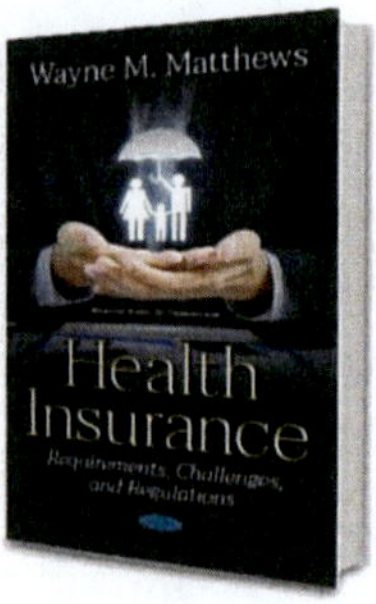

EDITOR: Wayne M. Matthews

SERIES: Health Care in Transition

BOOK DESCRIPTION: Since January 1, 2014, most individuals have had to maintain health insurance coverage or pay a penalty for noncompliance implemented through the Internal Revenue Code (IRC).

HARDCOVER ISBN: 978-1-53614-935-7
RETAIL PRICE: $195